DO NOT REMOVE
CARDS FROM POCKET

ALLEN COUNTY PUBLIC LIBRARY

FORT WAYNE, INDIANA 46802

You may return this book to any agency, branch,
or bookmobile of the Allen County Public Library.

DEMCO

ONE MONTH LIGHTER

ONE MONTH LIGHTER

TONI MAROTTA
LOLLY WURTZEL
— with —
Ruth Winter

A Stonesong Press Book

Arbor House/New York

Designed by Rueith Ottiger/Levavi & Levavi

Manufactured in the United States of America

10   9   8   7   6   5   4   3   2   1

This book is printed on acid free paper. The paper in this book meets the guidelines for permanence and durability of the Committee on Production Guidelines for Book Longevity of the Council on Library Resources.

Library of Congress Cataloging in Publication Data

Marotta, Antonia S.
   One month lighter.

   "A Stonesong Press book."
   Includes index.
   1. Reducing diets. 2. Reducing diets—Recipes.
I. Wurtzel, Lorraine Fay. II. Winter, Ruth, 1930–
III. Title.
RM222.2.M3616   1985   613.2′5   85-1296

ISBN 0-87795-671-5

———

To all the supportive

and loving family of staff

and members who make up

the Dynamic called Lean Line

Contents

Foreword

The Lean Line Program, now one of the most successful and popular diet regimens in America, was first developed in 1968 by Toni Marotta and Lolly Wurtzel with the professional advice of Arnold Lazarus, Ph.D., professor of psychology in the Graduate School of Applied and Professional Psychology at Rutgers University, and myself. Since then, more than a million people have found the Lean Line method unique, safe and easy to follow.

When I first met Lolly Wurtzel and Toni Marotta, I didn't know if I could trust them. I wasn't sure how serious they were about wanting to develop this diet. I didn't know how much advice they would accept.

They were serious. They did and do follow expert advice, and the Lean Line Program today is a very positive one. It is not only good for those who want to lose weight but for those who want to follow a healthy diet.

The Lean Line Program, because it is nutritionally sound, allows you to be in good shape metabolically. Thus, you will not suffer the psychological stresses that most diets cause. You will also avoid psychological stress, because the Lean Line program is much more in tune than most diets with what an individual likes to eat. So many other diet programs are simply a long list of foods you are not supposed to have, a common trap for those who attempt to stay on a regimen. The Lean Line Program provides the widest possible selection and, with very few exceptions, avoids total exclusion of any foods. Therefore, it eliminates the frustration, anger, and annoyance that are involved with the majority of weight-loss efforts.

On the Lean Line Program you will almost certainly eat a greater variety of foods than you have been eating. Most people become accustomed to just a few menu choices. Variety is essential. On the one hand, no one food provides all the nutrients needed, and on the other, there are some harmful components naturally present in almost all foods available to us, and overeating one such food can be damaging. For example, a person with thyroid problems should avoid eating too much cabbage, which contains a natural ingredient that binds with the thyroid hormone. Also good to keep in mind is that a great many vegetables contain compounds that inactivate vitamin B_1. But the quantity of these substances present in most vegetables is generally small, and their potency depends on the particular vegetable and the amount eaten. Thus, there is normally no need for alarm, since we generally do not consume enough of any one vegetable to cause problems. By having a variety of foods, you are assured that you will get enough of the nutrients necessary and very little of any particular harmful ingredient that may be hidden in the food.

In addition to offering great variety, including ethnic favorites, the Lean Line Program helps you learn new eating behaviors. The question is often asked, Why do so many of us have difficulty controlling food intake and end up overeating?

Scientists have been studying the factors that control food intake for a long time. Once it was believed that the blood glucose level was the major controlling factor that triggered hunger or appetite; when several hours after a meal the blood sugar level decreased, our hunger or appetite centers aroused us to the point that we would eat again. Today, we know that this is a highly simplistic answer to a complex question. No doubt blood glucose levels are important, but from a strictly practical point of view, you must take three factors into account:

1. Your caloric needs. The more calories you need in the conduct of your daily activities, the greater your appetite will be.

2. The bulk and volume of the foods you eat. Feelings of satiation are brought on through the filling of your intestinal tract by food. If you eat foods that are highly concentrated, which means they supply little if any fiber, you will tend to overeat even though your caloric needs have been met. Your needs for bulk will not have been met until you have overconsumed the concentrated foods and therefore are well on your way to obesity because of a lack of sufficient bulk or fiber in your diet. On the other hand, it is possible but rare for a person to eat foods so high in bulk that the caloric needs are not met. Such a person eventually would have nutritional deficiencies.

A balanced diet is one that provides the daily caloric and other nutritional needs with a minimum of refined sugar and the right amount of bulk or fiber so that you will not overeat or be undernourished. In short, a balanced diet provides the essential nutrients our bodies need.

Less obvious are the beneficial effects of certain foods that have become known only in the last few years. Present in cereals and in many fruits and vegetables are a group of compounds best identified as complex carbohydrates. These compounds include pectins, various vegetable gums, and carrageenan, which is derived from seaweed. Some of these substances you have no doubt heard about or even used. Pectin, for example, is used in making jams and jellies. Carrageenan and various gums are used to improve the texture of dairy products, such as cream cheese and artificial sour cream. However, they are usually used in small amounts in such processed foods.

Since these materials provide a certain amount of bulk in our diets, they aid in the proper movement of the intestinal tract, which in turn helps to regulate food intake, digestion, and absorption of nutrients. In addition, it has been found that guar gum, pectin, and carrageenan reduce the absorption of fat in the foods we eat, including cholesterol. Thus, pectin in our diets can prevent the utilization of some of the fat, including cholesterol, that we may normally ingest with various foods, such as eggs, butter, and meat. It has long been known that pectin is also an excellent detoxifying agent in the digestive tract and can prevent the absorption of heavy metals that may contaminate food. The Lean Line Program includes plenty of foods with pectin and vegetable gums.

There are many other substances present in foods that have not yet been studied under exacting conditions. It is surprising that after many decades of nutrition research so very little is known about the interplay of nutrition, taste, and smell and their respective roles in affecting the kinds and amounts of foods we eat.

3. Your consumption of refined sugar or sucrose. If you consume too much refined sugar, which provides only calories and has no nutrients and fiber, you stimulate your taste buds, and during a lifetime of eating foods high in sugar, you can develop cravings for sweet-tasting things, creating a desire for candy, cakes, and other such foods far beyond that which a person who does not normally consume much refined sugar will have. Therefore, it is particularly important that young children be kept away from highly sugared foods as much as possible. Early exposure to products such as soda, candy, baked goods usually leads to the development of a sweet tooth—a great need to satisfy sensations associated with the taste of sweetness.

We often tend to buy foods that are high in taste but low in nutrition. Does our body tell us when to stop eating foods that are nutritionally inadequate or downright harmful? In the case of experimental animals, we do know that they will reject very quickly a diet that is lacking in an essential vitamin or amino acid. However, we also observed that we can sometimes "fool" the animal by cloaking an inadequate diet with sugar. The animal will disregard its natural choice of a diet that is nutritious and choose the sweet stuff up to a point. After that, it will stop consuming sugar and again choose the nutritious diet if it is available.

Do we have a similar control mechanism that will make us stop after consuming large amounts of sweets that contribute little in the way of required nutrients? There is some indirect evidence that we do. Most of us have had the experience of tiring very quickly of eating excessive amounts of candy or sweet pastry, even if we normally enjoy such food. This observation is particularly striking when we compare it to the consumption of an unusually bland food—bread. Most populations throughout the world consume bread in one form or another and never tire of it despite the fact that it is eaten day in and day out, usually several times a day. This is in sharp contrast to the foods with a high sugar content. Unfortunately, sugary foods are packed with calories, and even though you may get sick of eating them quite quickly, they just as quickly add weight to your body.

On the subject of blood sugar, individuals who decide on their own, without medical supervision, to attempt to reduce their body weight by total starvation can incur a hypoglycemic state, a condition of very low blood sugar that can lead to cold sweat, trembling, and other undesirable symptoms. There are a great many situations that can lead to a reduction in blood sugar, including drinking too much alcohol and eating extremely high-protein meals, both of which affect the production of insulin, the hormone that reduces blood sugar levels. Another important cause of low blood sugar is prolonged starvation. Skipping breakfast, a common habit of many persons attempting to lose weight, can also cause hypoglycemic symptoms. If your last meal of the day is consumed somewhere around 6 P.M., even if an additional snack is consumed later at night, eight to ten hours will elapse before you normally consume breakfast. If you skip breakfast, twelve to fourteen hours will have elapsed between meals. This is an inordinately long time interval and can lead to low blood sugar. If you expect to carry out your activities with alertness, without excessive fatigue, then you must ingest nutrients at regular intervals. Also, by providing the body with an excess of nutrients all at once, say at dinner time only, the cells and organs will find it difficult to cope with the excess, and erratic metabolism will result.

Excessive exercise or overly strenuous exertion can also lead to hypoglycemic symptoms. Usually, however, these symptoms will pass as the cause is removed. True hypoglycemia, which is rare, can only be substantiated by a carefully supervised glucose tolerance test. The common symptoms of low blood sugar that so many dieters on unbalanced programs experience constitute no major cause for alarm. What these symptoms point out, however, is that any type of diet program, whether it includes weight control, reduction of food intake, or exercise, needs to be done in moderation and with the advice of experts.

The Lean Line Program has incorporated into a healthy, workable plan the three major aspects of weight control:

1. the amount of calories consumed,

2. a moderate exercise program, and

3. help in coping with the emotional difficulties and tensions of achieving and maintaining proper body weight.

No matter how much a person might wish to hide behind such vague notions as endocrine problems, or other abnormal metabolism problems, the simple fact remains that body weight is a reflection of the total number of calories consumed minus the number of calories expended in the form of physical activity or exercise. Having an awareness of the total calories consumed in one day is essential.

There is a good deal of confusion and some hype about the value of exercise for people who want to lose weight. The truth is the role of exercise in relation to *weight control* is relatively minor. The number of calories expended during a half hour or even one hour of relatively heavy activity does not add up to many slices of bread or, God forbid, even a small piece of cake or a bowl of ice cream. However, there are benefits, the most important of which is the beneficial effect of exercise on the body's circulation, which in very basic terms means the transport of life-essential oxygen and other nutrients to all the cells, tissues, and organs of the body. There is no question that good circulation obtained through a good exercise program leads to better health—both mental and physical. An interesting aspect of exercise is that not only will it usually not increase one's appetite, it may even curb it. Therefore, whatever calories are used up are a kind of bonus.

What kind of exercise is best for those on a Lean Line Program? The choice is up to you, but I like a brisk twenty-minute walk each day or a swim. Most physicians and psychologists recommend vigorous exercise for about half an hour a day at least three times a week. Such exercises are aerobic, that is, they increase oxygen consumption and burn calories rapidly. Tennis, golf, and jogging have their drawbacks because they overemploy a few muscles. Walking and swimming, on the other hand, are better because they are aerobic, use the muscles of the entire body, and do not overstress certain muscles and joints.

As for the third major aspect of weight loss, *help,* all of us need someone on whose shoulder we can lean and perhaps occasionally cry. Such support is particularly valuable when trying to control weight. One of the reasons for the great success of Lean Line is the support the group and its personnel provide. But if you cannot get to a Lean Line Program, a spouse, relative, or friend can provide support and understanding when needed. And, more important, you now have this book.

The Lean Line Program has a vast array of permitted foods in all categories. If you follow the One Month Lighter Program, you will lose weight and learn a lot about proper eating. After four weeks, when you set up your own diet program continuing to use what you have learned, you should also make a real effort to expand the number of foods in your daily menu and not just select the relatively few foods that you like or that you have limited yourself to for years. You now have the opportunity to follow a nutritionally and psychologically sound diet program that has been successful for thousands of people and can be successful for you. There are no gimmicks and no false promises. There is, however, a great opportunity to change the way you eat, feel, and look.

> Dr. Hans Fisher
> Chairman, Department of Nutrition
> Rutgers University

PART I

LOSING 15 TO 20 POUNDS IN JUST ONE MONTH

1. HOW IT ALL BEGAN . . . AND WHY IT WORKS

When my third son was christened, I, Toni Marotta, baked cookies. So many cookies, in fact, that the leftovers filled a dozen five-quart jars. My husband worked late in those days, so I spent many evenings alone after our kids had gone to bed. It didn't take me more than a few nights to empty those cookie jars.

Chocolate was my downfall. I'm Lolly Wurtzel, and I put a many-pocketed apron my mother-in-law gave me to good use. I put a can of chocolate syrup in one pocket and straws in the other and in between house-cleaning chores and caring for the kids, I'd take a straw, put it in the can, and sip the chocolate.

Our stories are not too different from those of our members: Sally, for example, rescued brownies from the garbage can and ate them, and John, our secret eater, in terror of his wife discovering his bathroom eating habits, hid a gallon of ice cream in the hamper and forgot about it.

We are sure you have your own story to tell, as do the thousands of others who come to us wanting to be thin, each of whom had once expected to end life's frustrations and celebrate its joys at the bottom of a can of chocolate syrup or a jar of cookies. They did not recognize the sad irony that those frustrations actually began with the foods they sought solace in. Hence arose the thousands of diet clubs, spas, diets, diet plans, diet foods, all wonderful, helpful—and mostly unsuccessful. We will not depress you with the statistics showing how few actually make it.

If you are a dieter, you are most likely among the ranks of the disenchanted. This program may seem like just another grand promise of success, and you've been down that road enough times to feel that the Lean Line Program probably won't work either. We understand your despair but nevertheless invite you to abandon once more the justifiable disenchantment of the jaded dieter and consider the following: There *are* people who *do* make it to the finish line (goal weight) and are able to permanently control their weight. What do these people know or do that evades the majority? We can give you the answer.

We met in 1968. At that time, Lolly was a lecturer for a diet group after having gone through the program. Toni was an attendee. The group program worked well. Most do. We trimmed down. But after finishing the course, to our dismay, we both began to put on the pounds again.

We both had battled a weight problem all of our lives. We asked ourselves, Why can't we stay thin? We were alike and yet we were different. Toni was Italian and Lolly was Jewish. Toni associated family feasts with lasagna and meatballs and spaghetti. Lolly remembered happy Sunday mornings with Grandma and cousins and lox and bagels. Our ethnic foods were part of who we were. How could we keep to a diet without them? The urge would overcome us. We would go back to eating the foods we loved, feel guilty, and another diet would be gone. There had to be a different way. We found it. We consulted Dr. Hans Fisher, chairman of the Department of Food Science at Rutgers University, and Dr. Arnold Lazarus, professor of psychology at the Rutgers Graduate School of Clinical and Applied Psychology. The resulting Lean Line Program represents eighty years of combined experience in the weight-reduction field.

Our regimen is based on balanced calories and psychological techniques. We know there is so much more to losing weight than a decision to cut out certain foods or reduce total food intake. The groundwork takes place in the one part of your body that doesn't have a weight problem—your brain. The Lean Line approach was an immediate success because it represents a breakthrough in dieting.

We scraped together $300 from our savings and rented a dilapidated hall in Colonia, N.J., and ran a little classified ad in the local paper. We were delighted when ten women showed up for the first meeting. Today, our business grosses more than $1 million a year. It includes Lean Line business in eight states; Lean Line diet foods, including a low-calorie Italian sausage; Lean Line diet dens, which sell calorie-controlled products; and centers serving persons with weight problems requiring close medical supervision. We employ more than 300 people. At least 1.5 million people have lost weight on the Lean Line Program—and have kept it off.

There are many reasons we have been so successful with "seasoned dieters," who have lost and gained and lost and gained again and again on every other imaginable diet regimen. Our program not only takes into consideration ethnic foods—anyone's ethnic foods—but it provides insight into what triggers your eating. Do you eat, for example, when you are happy? Sad? When your husband comes home late from work? When the kids frustrate you?

The insight makes it possible to avoid automatic eating

and gives you a choice. You can have your ethnic foods and other foods you love as long as you know why you want to eat them, and eat them in proper proportions. There are some foods that have to be handled carefully, such as liquor and pie à la mode, but even they may be incorporated into your diet.

With the Lean Line Program, we were finally able to lose weight ourselves and to keep it off. And we've helped people from all walks of life. One was a nun who came to us when her order changed from habits to civilian dress and she could no longer hide her girth beneath flowing robes; the Lean Line Program changed her other "habits" as well. Another was a chef in a famous restaurant who did more than taste the tempting dishes he created. The program we have developed works not only because it is nutritionally and psychologically sound but because it emphasizes eating the foods you love.

We have a weight-loss program, not a diet. A program connotes change, while a diet connotes sacrifice. With the Lean Line Program:

I You do not have to punish yourself to lose weight.
I You do not have to deny yourself your favorite foods.
I You can enjoy your meals at home, at work, and in a restaurant.
I You can succeed in taking off weight and keeping it off, even if many times before you have failed—and you probably have.

We recently had one woman who came to us and said that she'd love to lose her ten extra pounds but she could "never stick to a diet." She said she had tried every book and every diet that came along, and each time she'd lose five or six pounds and then go on an eating binge and gain all the weight back. "I just don't have enough motivation to stick it out," she said with a sigh.

We pointed out to her that when she took into consideration all her various diets, she'd find she had really lost more than 250 pounds.

Now, that takes willpower. Anyone who can diet away the same old five or ten or twenty pounds time after time must have enormous desire, self-discipline, and perseverance. People who can grimly pit themselves against pizza and fudge for weeks at a time have enough willpower for any army.

Then why is this woman who lost more than 250 pounds still 10 pounds overweight? Because she *thinks* like a fat person, and dieting is what fat folks do—over and over again.

The Lean Line Program has been heralded in recent years as a miracle diet. There are no miracle diets and no miracle foods! What has been interpreted as the Lean Line miracle diet is actually a formula expressing the results of a study of successful dieters and the techniques they had in common. This formula was turned into a simple usable method of losing weight and keeping it off. It has been used consistently and successfully by people who up to now have failed.

If you follow the Lean Line One Month Lighter Program described in Chapter 4, you will not only shed pounds, you will have fun, you will not be hungry, and you will feel better and have more energy than you've had in years. And perhaps, most important of all, by the end of the month, you will have learned how effortless it is to think and eat like a healthy, thin person.

We've made it easy for you. All the foods are available in your local market, and many are probably on your pantry shelf. In the first part of the One Month Lighter Program, we've included every meal and snack in a safe, nutritious, and delicious program. You will lose weight on the plan and be comforted by the fact that you're eating a delicious and varied menu that allows for your own personal preferences.

In Chapter 9 we show you how to set up your own diet program, and in Part II we provide many additional wholemeal recipes. You can substitute dishes you prefer on any day in either the program we've set up or the one you are going to follow on your own. The substitutions, of course, should be equivalent, using, for example, one vegetable dish instead of another or one protein dish, such as fish, instead of veal. Our program emphasizes choices, but there are some things that you must do to make it work for you.

There are *six* basic food lists from which you will be selecting your food intake for the day: Protein, Vegetable, Bread, Milk, Fruit, and Oil and Condiment lists. There are also two Bonus Lists, but items on it are not required. Nutritional requirements differ for men, women, and preteens, and that is taken into account. See the lists in Chapter 9.

There's no guilt with this program. Toni still eats her favorite lasagna, and Lolly, her lox and bagels. You can eat apple pie, ice cream, spaghetti, and pizza (see pages 229–33). We teach you how to "decalorize" any dish. We teach you moderation. And, if you do slip, so what? That doesn't make you a failure or a bad person. It makes you human. Just get yourself back on track. Eventually, you won't slip, because eating like a thin person will become a habit.

If you follow the One Month Lighter Program and then create your own Lean Line Program, you will not only learn a lot about proper nutrition, you will learn a lot about yourself. You'll suddenly realize you are not different from your size-five neighbor or your thin sibling. It's just that your body's internal computer has been programmed incorrectly. Its instructions have led you to overeat or to eat the wrong foods. You will develop a new set of instructions in your personal file to call up when you are faced with a choice of foods.

You can't design a new program for yourself, however, until you know something about your old program. You have to "read it" so that you know where the glitches are.

We help you do that by helping you understand your BASIC ID (see Chapter 2).

With your inner computer programmed properly, you'll be able to go into a restaurant and eat just like anyone else. You can have lunch with a business associate and he or she will never even be aware that you are keeping track of calories.

When you're upset, you will no longer stuff your mouth for comfort. Lolly remembers the time, for example, when she was at the beach with her husband and one of her young sons. "My husband thought he was being funny when he said to our son as he was about to follow me into the water, 'Don't go in. Your mother is using the ocean.' I laughed with everyone else, but then I went and ate three hamburgers at the food stand."

If your spouse or a relative or friend tempts you, you'll understand it's their problem, not yours, and forgive them.

"My mother was a real old-fashioned mama," Toni recalls. "If you didn't eat when she offered you food, you were either sick or didn't love her."

We'll give you hints that are fun and will go far in helping you reprogram yourself: eating with chopsticks, for example, or using a pickle fork instead of a regular one. See if that doesn't slow you down. And how about wearing white gloves when you go to a party? Did you ever try picking up fattening food—or any food—with clean white gloves?

One of the cornerstones of our program is helping people express their anger instead of "eating it." We have been partners for more than sixteen years, but once in a while we get angry at each other. We share the same office. Sometimes we scare newly hired secretaries when they listen to the yelling coming from our office, but everyone at Lean Line headquarters in South Plainfield, N.J., soon realizes that not only are we the best of friends but we also care deeply about the organization. Both of us get the greatest thrill from seeing people who before could never successfully stick to a weight-loss program succeed with ours.

When you read this book and follow the Lean Line Program for just *one month,* we promise you you'll not only be lighter,

- You will be richer because the healthy foods in the program are less expensive than the sweet fattening foods you usually eat.
- You will have reprogrammed your inner computer, and wise eating will become automatic.
- You will feel better physically.
- You will feel more in control of your life.
- You will know *how to be a thin person for life.*

2. YOUR BASIC ID: UNDERSTANDING YOUR INTERNAL PROGRAMMING

Most people aren't really aware of why they eat the way they do; sometimes the effect of their weight loss on their personality can be quite unexpected. Beneath the fat, there is always a complicated person.

Janice, for example, never thought of herself as being overweight. "I was a size five when I married, and in my mind, I was still a size five, even though I wore a size twenty-two and a half, and that was tight," the five foot one, former 265 pounder recalls. "Still, I liked myself and I had a lot of friends because I was very outgoing and 'jolly,' like fat people are supposed to be.

"My husband, Bill, never said a word about my being overweight. Just once, I saw a woman on the street and said,

'Look, she's fatter than I am,' and he said, 'No, she's not!'

"A group of women from the PTA were going to go to Lean Line and they said, 'Hey, you're fatter than any of us. Why don't you come with us?' I figured I had nothing else social to do at night, so I decided to go with them.

"I guess, underneath, I really wanted to lose weight. My friends from the PTA lost three pounds the first week. I didn't. I was very discouraged, and the next week I lost a quarter of a pound. I had tears in my eyes, but the Lean Line lecturer was most supportive, and she urged me to stick with it. The third week, I lost seven pounds and the next, five. It was a lot of water weight at first, but once I started to lose, I kept losing. I lost one hundred and twenty-eight pounds all together and I've kept them off for two years.

"My husband and son joined Lean Line six months ago on their own, and they are managing their own programs. My son wanted to make the basketball team, but he was too heavy. He still was too heavy at the end of the school year but the coach so admired his effort that he promised him in the fall he would put him on the team."

Janice, who has large blue eyes and straight brown hair, talks animatedly but is really quite shy.

"I had a funny reaction after I lost weight. I became much quieter, and it was harder for me to socialize with people. I think I was hiding behind the fat. Now that people can see the real me, I feel sort of exposed. But I'm working on it. And the fact that I was able to control my diet had a positive effect on my sense of competence. I've gone back and finished college, and now I'm in a master's program in social work. I don't think I would have taken the challenge of going back to school before."

We think of Janice and other overweight people as buried treasure—a chest filled with diamonds. The diamonds are buried not in earth but in fat, and we provide the tools to dig out the diamonds—the thin, sparkling individual.

Take Soni. Her weight loss was not as dramatic as Janice's, but the results were. Soni was a forty-two-year-old housewife who had emigrated from Scandinavia at the age of sixteen. She had let her blond hair turn stringy gray, wore shapeless dresses and no makeup, and had put on an extra twenty-five pounds since her marriage. When she lost weight on the Lean Line Program, she had her hair restyled and colored, bought new dresses, and made herself very attractive. She obtained a job as a sales representative and is now very successful.

"Sometimes," she confides, "I still feel like that awkward sixteen-year-old immigrant inside, and then I look in the mirror and see a confident, slim, American career woman."

What do you see when you look in the mirror? It doesn't matter how others see you. It is your self-image that counts.

Our Lean Line consultant Dr. Arnold Lazarus emphasizes that it is not what happens to us but our perceptions, beliefs, and what we tell ourselves about what happens to us that produce stressful emotions and cause almost all forms of emotional distress. "We react to our perceptions of the world, not the world itself," he says.

Do you see yourself as a fat or thin person when you look in the mirror? Are you good-looking or dowdy? Happy or angry? It is the image of yourself that *you* see that counts.

You have your own reasons for gaining weight. They may not be the same as Janice's or Soni's or your friends or those of the person sitting next to you on the bus. That's why there is no single solution to a weight problem, and what works for someone else may not work for you.

In order to succeed in losing pounds and keeping them off, you have to understand what's really behind your own personal eating behavior. All too frequently, we blame our emotions for our lack of success on a diet. We use them like a crutch, saying, "I was so angry, I ate everything in sight" or "When things aren't going right and I feel down, I go off my diet."

Emotions are a normal part of living, and the key to success in staying on a program is learning how to separate our *eating life* from our *emotional life.*

How do you act when you are angry? Do you suppress your anger? What do you do when someone hurts you? Do you automatically retreat into a shell? Do you automatically assume you are wrong? How do you know what makes you happy? Do you feel happy more than you feel angry, hurt, or depressed? How do you know when you are happy?

Dr. Lazarus, the founder of various multimodal therapy institutes, has helped us develop the BASIC ID part of our program. BASIC ID stands for Behavior, Affect, Sensation, Imagery, Cognition, Interpersonal, and Diet. Dr. Lazarus points out that Lean Line is the only major weight-loss program that uses the multimodal theory, which is built on the premise that "unless people are trained to deal with certain problems, many stones are left unturned. Problems will arise from under those stones and relapses will certainly ensue. The more coping responses you develop for overeating, the less likely you will suffer a relapse. Other weight-control programs may have behavior modification, but ours includes introspection as well. You've got to understand what your problem really is before you can learn behaviors with which to cope. Instead of just telling you to change your behavior, we say change your attitude toward emotions. Change your sensations. Change your images. Change your cognition. Change the way you deal with other people."

If you follow the BASIC ID that Dr. Lazarus helped us develop and think carefully about your answers, you may be able to discover for yourself why you overeat or eat the wrong things. You can make a connection between your childhood memories of discipline, pain, reward, and joy and how you eat. There are no right or wrong responses, only your own.

The first step toward the changes you can make is to understand the seven parts that make up your personality. They are:

1. *Behavior.* Behavior is how you act, what you do consciously or unconsciously. Conscious behavior requires thought. If you go out on the weekend and deliberately go off your diet, that's conscious. If you taste foods while cooking, that's unconscious behavior. Unconscious behavior is habit; no thought is involved. Eating is often impulsive. We love to tell the story about a member who was on one of her many diets, mainly cottage cheese and lettuce. She was sitting at a table in the plant cafeteria when she saw that a man had left two bran muffins on his tray. She reached over, grabbed the muffins, and gobbled them down. The man returned to the table with the butter he had forgotten for his muffins. After that she learned to control her impulses and changed her eating behavior. You can, too, if you pay attention to your eating behavior.

2. *Affect.* A fancy word for emotions, "affect" includes all of them—anger, love, depression, happiness. Many people associate food with love and comfort. Eating is often a way of dealing with emotional reactions. Karen not only ate when she was frustrated, she ate when she was happy. Since she was either frustrated or happy, she put on thirty pounds in her senior year of high school. After she joined Lean Line, Karen became aware of the fact that in her family food was used as a balm for any hurt. She learned to separate physical hunger from emotional hunger. She was slim and confident by the time she reached freshman orientation in college. We at Lean Line make every effort to help people separate emotions and eating.

3. *Sensation.* You have five senses: sight, hearing, smell, taste, and touch. If you are overweight, chances are you derive most of your sensual pleasures from taste. But when you think about it, you have just a small area of taste buds on your tongue, and those buds can only really identify sweet, sour, bitter, and salt. Smell also triggers eating. What could be more American than the scent of apple pie emanating from the kitchen? Odors can unconsciously trigger desire to eat because they remind us of foods from the past. Food should be terrific and "feed our senses." Our recipes—both plain and gourmet—feed our senses, but just because they taste, look, and smell good doesn't mean they are fattening. More important, tasting food should not be your only sensual pleasure. You have to start considering some of the others—touching someone you love, listening to music, seeing beautiful scenery, smelling salty air or a new perfume. If you fill your life with sensory experiences you won't rely on food for your only delight.

4. *Imagery.* You have the ability to picture something in your mind. Imagery can be useful in helping you "see" what you will look like when you are thin. Your imagination can also be used to change behavior. Anticipation is using your imagination to predict a coming event. Anticipation is wonderful. Sometimes, it's even better than the "real thing." The mind has incredible powers of creation; it feeds on old memories and future delights. You can use that power. For example, brochures make Hawaiian luaus seem romantic, with lit torches, girls in grass skirts, and a feast fit for a king. Your mind tells you that this is a gourmet experience not to be missed. The reality is something else—greasy pork, sodden vegetables, horrid tropical drinks tasting like sweet colored water. The delightful vision has been destroyed by the reality. You eat the food anyway. But if you can "imagine" behaving in an appropriate manner—not eating the greasy pork, for example—it is very likely you will behave in that manner. You can use your imagination for positive images, such as picturing yourself slim in a bathing suit or getting compliments from people as you are losing weight. You can also use negative images to help you resist. One Lean Line lecturer holds up a pound of chicken fat in a plastic bag and says, "Do you want to carry this around on your hips?" That works well. Or if you are really tempted, then just imagine poison or roaches on the food. That imagery really kills desire.

5. *Cognition.* Cognition is what you think and believe. Many beliefs you have about losing weight and keeping it off are erroneous or you wouldn't need this book. You believe, for example, that you can lose weight but not keep it off. You believe you can lose only a certain amount of weight. Your beliefs can be changed.

6. *Interpersonal.* "Interpersonal" refers to how you relate to other people. The key component in the Lean Line Program is learning how to assert yourself—to ask for and get what you want. Instead of expressing your anger or frustration by saying what is on your mind and taking appropriate action, you eat. It's not unlike the alcoholic who must have a drink when under stress or the smoker who must have a cigarette. Things we get off our chest should not end up on our hips.

7. *Diet.* This deals with your physiological being. It includes what you eat and how much you eat. It also encompasses health problems, such as high blood pressure and diabetes, and such factors as too little rest or exercise, too much stress, or poor metabolic rate.

Now, here is how you use the BASIC ID to help you succeed with the program. We at Lean Line firmly believe that the smartest place to start a diet is in your head. Let's take some typical problem (chances are, it's one of yours).

"When I get upset with someone who means a lot to me, I'd rather eat than say what is really bothering me."

The Problem	The Solution
Behavior—Overeating.	Behavior—I can perform various acts that interfere with overeating, such as taking a walk or going shopping (but not for food).

Affect—I don't cope well with anger. I tend to cover up feelings.

Affect—I will recognize that it is all right to feel anger. I will express feeling assertively but not aggressively.

Sensation—I feel tense and have butterflies in my stomach.

Sensation—I will practice relaxation and abdominal breathing exercises.

Imagery—I can't see myself being assertive.

Imagery—I will imagine myself talking out problems and finding solutions.

Cognition—I believe anger is not the correct response, so I suppress my anger and eat instead.

Cognition—It's all right to feel angry. I believe I can show how I feel. My opinions are valuable.

Interpersonal—I avoid expressing my feelings.

Interpersonal—I will write down how I feel. I will communicate my feelings directly to the person involved.

Diet—My eating rides alongside my anger

Diet—I will recognize that vigorous exercise will reduce my pent up anger.

"When I go to a family gathering, I get tempted and say, 'Oh, I love that, but I am going to eat just a little bit,' and I wind up eating every bit."

The Problem	The Solution
Behavior—Eatiing foods because they are available.	Behavior—I will preplan. I will eat something before I go. I have a choice of foods that I can eat and still stay on the program.
Affect—I'm anxious about being around old favorite foods and old relationships.	Affect—I'm happy to see my family. I can relax and enjoy the gathering.
Sensation—Sight and aroma of foods. Remembering the taste of these foods.	Sensation—I will shift the emphasis from food to the atmosphere. I will enjoy listening to the conversation.
Imagery—Playing the old tape of how I act when all the old favorite foods are around.	Imagery—I will reprogram the tape to show myself enjoying the food without going off the program. I can see myself eating only acceptable foods.
Cognition—I can't stay on a program when there are so many favorite foods available. I believe it is impossible to stay on a program at a family dinner.	Cognition—I will begin to believe it's important to stay on the program no matter what the circumstances. I can enjoy myself and lose weight.

Interpersonal—I feel the
       need to eat in
       family situa-
       tions.

Interpersonal—I will recog-
       nize that fam-
       ily situations
       and overeat-
       ing have no
       connection.

Diet—Doesn't allow me to
       eat when I go to a
       family party.

Diet—Since I am on a sensi-
       ble eating program, I
       have a great variety of
       foods from which to
       choose.

Now, write in your own worst problem with food and try to solve it:

The Problem

Behavior—I eat when I _____
_____.

The Solution

Behavior—I could, instead,
       behave differently.
       I could _____
       _____.

Affect—When I feel _____,
       I _____
       _____.

Affect—If I could _____,
       I could feel _____
       _____.

Sensation—When my _____,
       I feel _____
       _____.

Sensation—I could change
       that by concen-
       trating on my
       sense of _____.
       I will enjoy _____
       instead.

Imagery—I can't see myself
       _____.

Imagery—I can imagine my-
       self _____
       _____.

Cognition—I believe I
       shouldn't_____.
       I believe I can't
       _____.

Cognition—Actually, I really
       don't have to ___.
       I can _____
       _____.

Interpersonal—I can't communicate to
_____

that I _____.

Interpersonal—Here's how
I really feel
_____

and I'm going
to express
the fact that

_____.

Diet—I always eat too much
when_____
_____.

Diet—Instead of eating I can
_____

and feel good about
staying on the Lean
Line Program.

Once you have practiced analyzing your problem, you can deal with your behavior. As Dr. Lazarus points out, when negative events occur, it is normal to feel annoyed, frustrated, or irritated, but you should not be totally racked with disgust or dread or terror. So you need to make a conscious effort to stop using such words as "dreadful," "awful," "terrible," and "disgusting" about yourself and your behavior and substitute such words as "inconvenient," "frustrating," "annoying," and "irritating."

If you change your vocabulary it will help you gain control of your negative feelings. If you do this consistently, you will feel much better about yourself, and this, in turn, will make it easier for you to control your negative feelings and impulses.

Instead of thinking, feeling, and saying, "I should," "I must," or "I have to" about your personal decisions and choices, train yourself instead to think, feel, and say, "I would prefer" or "It would be better to."

By changing such negative ways of expressing yourself, you won't feel resentful that something has been imposed on you. You will feel as if this change in your eating habits is something you *want* to accomplish. If you pressure yourself into an impossible situation by telling yourself, "I have to lose two pounds this week," and you only lose one and a half pounds, you will feel like a failure. If you say, "I would prefer to lose two pounds this week," and you don't, you can say, "Well, maybe next week." It takes the pressure off.

The Lean Line emphasis on choices concerns more than what and how much you eat: You can choose to be thin. Take a pencil and paper and write down on one side of the paper the advantages of staying as you are now, and on the other side, the advantages of losing weight and being slim.

Some of the advantages of being overweight are that you can eat as much as you want of fattening foods, feel comforted by gorging on sweets, and feel virtuous by leaving your plate clean as you did when you were a child. You can wear tent dresses or baggy pants and sit on wide-bottomed chairs and protect yourself from an active social and sexual life. You will always have an excuse for any rejection: "I'm overweight."

Some of the advantages of being slim include being able to cross your legs, looking great in clothes, dancing, swimming, feeling sexy, looking younger. Thin means belts, bikinis, boots, and really tasting and enjoying food, perhaps for the first time.

If you think about it, the key ingredient to any success—not just in controlling your weight—is the ability to motivate yourself. Of course, you've heard that before, but how can you motivate yourself to stick to the Lean Line Program? Ask yourself the following basic questions:

∎ Can it be done?
∎ Is it worth the effort?
∎ What is my alternative?

If you answer yes to the first two, you're on your way. If you answer no, consider the alternative.

Today is the first day of the rest of your life. Is today the day you are going to begin loving and respecting yourself enough to use the tools we offer so that you will be able to see the real you in the mirror a month from now?

QUESTIONS TO TEST YOUR COGNITION ABOUT DIETING
Answer True or False and then see the answers below.

1. Overweight people are easily stimulated by the sight and smell of food. _____

2. For many overweight people, there is a weight at which they get stuck and can't reduce further. _____

3. It is easier to maintain a low weight than it is to lose it. _____

4. Weekends are the most difficult time for many dieters. _____

5. Men lose weight faster than women. _____

6. Overweight people tend to lack assertiveness. _____

7. You shouldn't eat potatoes and bread the same day. _____

8. Overweight people are often jolly and happy. _____

9. You always lose weight when you are ill.

10. Pounds quickly gained are quickly lost.

11. It won't do any harm to binge if you cut back on what you eat the next day. _____

Answers to True-False Quiz

1. *True.* The overweight can easily be tempted to go off a diet when confronted by the sight, sound, or smell of food. TV commercials about food or walking through a supermarket are enough to provide the stimuli.

2. *True.* The problem is not a physical one but stems from the belief people have about a number. The belief may be rooted in past experience, or it may have evolved from other people telling dieters they already look good. If dieters can be encouraged to get below the number at which they are stuck, the barrier will be shattered and they can continue to lose weight.

3. *False.* It is more difficult to maintain a weight loss for several reasons. One reason is that once a goal is reached, the compliments and encouragement we get from others tend to wane. We also tend to believe that once we are thin, we can go back to our old eating habits. Our expectations of how being thin will change our lives are often unrealistic; they will not solve all our problems—only one of them.

4. *True.* For many overweight people, weekends are a time to go off a diet. This may be because it is what we have always done in the past—diet during the week and binge on the weekends. Another reason weekends can be a problem is that we have less of a routine and have more time to snack.

5. *True.* Men have a higher metabolic rate than women and consequently lose faster.

6. *True.* Overweight people have difficulty asking for what they want and getting it. They are often unable to say no in all life's situations in addition to food.

7. *False.* Potatoes are a vegetable, and a balanced diet includes both vegetables and breads. They are not nutritional equals.

8. *False.* The happy fat person is quite frequently a front for someone who has become the life of the party so as not to become the brunt of jokes.

9. *False.* It happens quite often that you gain weight when you are ill because you abandon a sound nutritional program. You rely on those foods that someone said would make you better, like chicken soup, fruit juices, and breads.

10. *False.* Every dieter has found that it takes longer to lose weight than it does to gain. Those three pounds gained in a weekend might take three weeks to take off.

11. *False.* You may have relied on the binge-and-starve syndrome as a weight-reduction method out of habit, not because it works. What usually happens is that while you are "starving," you become so hungry you overeat again.

3. SUREFIRE TIPS FOR LOSING WEIGHT THE LEAN LINE WAY

No one is too old, too young, or too set in his or her ways to lose weight successfully. You *can* lose weight safely and keep it off if you follow the One Month Lighter Program described in this book.

First of all, accept the fact that those extra pounds you are lugging around are a sign that you are burdened with a load of inappropriate eating habits. Somehow or other you picked up the behavior patterns of a fat person and made them your own. Now is the time to exchange them for the eating habits of a thin person. It really is simple to stop the automatic procedures you've been using and replace them with new ones.

▌ *Slow down.* The most common behavioral problem overweight people have is not their eating chocolate cake, it
is eating it too fast!

Your stomach is the slowest-acting organ in your
body. It takes about 20 minutes for it to signal your
brain that it has had enough. If you eat quickly, you can
eat a five-course meal and have "seconds" of everything
before your brain is notified that you've had too much.

Just by slowing down your eating—that simple behavior change alone—you will automatically eat less.

You can help yourself slow your intake by putting
down your fork between every bite, chewing your food
very well, and then swallowing it before picking up your
fork again. You can also use a pickle fork or chopsticks
to help slow you down. Keep a clock in front of you, if
necessary, to make sure that you take at least twenty
minutes to eat a meal.

If you slow down, you will savor your meal. Most
overweight people gulp their food without giving their
taste buds a chance to know what's coming through. We
ask you to enjoy eating by *concentrating on it.* Did you ever
sit in a restaurant next to a thin woman and really
watch her eat? She will probably select some dish you
think should be forbidden on a diet. Then she will eat it
slowly, while conversing, and savor every bite. She will
probably also leave a portion of it on the plate.

Slowing down your eating behavior is a cardinal rule
for sensible weight reduction; recording on paper your
intake is another.

▌ *Write down what you eat.* Since most overweight people eat
subconsciously and don't realize how much they really
ingest—all those little tastes of this and that—recording
intake on paper really helps. And besides, if your hand is
on the pencil, you'll think twice before putting it on the
fork. See the Food and Emotions Chart on page 74.

▌ *Eat at the same time every day.* Eat your meals at the same time each day by planning a twenty-four-hour schedule that suits you—and then stick to it. Eating at the same time each day will help you concentrate on your food, and it will give your body a chance to program its internal metabolic clock. Once you establish order, your body will tell you when it's time to eat—and it won't send out false alarms at all hours of the day and night. If a desire for food is triggered between mealtimes, remember that between-meal snacks can be part of your Lean Line Program. You have a wide variety of snacks you can select from the Free Food List (page 182) and Bonus Lists (pages 180 and 181), or you may save a dessert, bread, or milk selection from a meal so that you can eat it later. Snacks, however, like everything else, should be planned and eaten according to all Lean Line recommended techniques. For example, even an apple or orange should be put down between bites.

▌ *Eat in the same place.* Pick one place in your home—and if necessary one place in the cafeteria or lunch room at your job—and eat meals and snacks there. Restrict your eating places to as few as possible. No midnight snacks in bed, no nibbling in front of the TV. The fewer eating spots you have, the less often your desire to eat will be triggered. When you travel or dine out, of course, you won't be able to sit in your usual place; but you can simulate it by facing the same way you usually do or sit on the same side of the table.

▌ *Don't do anything else while eating.* At home or away, break old associations by cutting out all mealtime activities except talking. Give your mealtimes and snack times to the enjoyment of eating, and perhaps some pleasant conversation. Save reading, television watching, driving, sewing, and desk work for their own place and time. All of these activities trigger your old food-binge tapes.

▎ *Never eat standing up.* It is amazing how much food we can consume on the run—a quick doughnut while on the way to the office or a chunk of cheese in the kitchen while passing the refrigerator. We tend to think that what we eat while standing up somehow doesn't count—as though we didn't really eat that cookie, or perhaps all the calories magically leaked out of the bottom before it got into our mouths. If you sit down and eat it, you'll know you're eating, and you'll know you're not eating in your assigned place at the assigned time.

▎ *Use smaller plates and cutlery.* Stow away your dinner plates. Place your entrée on a salad plate and your salad in a saucer. Use a fruit-juice glass and a demitasse cup for beverages. Use a salad or shrimp fork, a demitasse spoon, and a butter knife for your silverware.

This simple change will take advantage of your ability to create optical illusions. Moreover, psychological research has demonstrated that the use of such optical illusions actually works to reduce food intake. All of us are stimulated by what we see, so that the way food looks on a plate helps determine how satisfying we find it. When we look at a plate of food, our inner computer automatically registers two things; amount and appearance. We determine the amount of food by how full or empty the plate looks. When we see a lonely scoop of tuna fish marooned on a tiny lettuce leaf in the middle of a large plate, we feel deprived before we even pick up the fork. But put the same quantity of food on a smaller plate, making the plate look fuller, and we will be satisfied. In one study, twenty dieters were asked to serve themselves on salad plates, while twenty others served themselves on dinner plates. Both groups were allotted the same amount of food. More than seventy percent of those who ate from salad plates reported that their satisfaction increased—even though they knew they were getting the same amount of food as those who ate from dinner plates.

Small serving dishes create the illusion of quantity that triggers satisfaction, and they actually hold less food. Thus, you can refill your plate with "seconds" and still be eating your "firsts."

Eating with small utensils also seems to make the food more satisfying by making it last longer, supporting the twenty-minute mealtime minimum.

Eye appeal and sensual satisfaction are vital to a successful weight-loss program. There is nothing visually appetizing about a limp, soggy salad, and even the prettiest vegetable is tedious when served on an ugly dish. Vary the texture and color of food; a firm white fish, a crisp green vegetable, and a succulent red tomato salad set on a pretty plate are not only eye filling but hunger satisfying as well. Your mind gets the message that what you are eating is not a tiresome sacrifice. To make the meal even more enjoyable—a real occasion—dress up the table with a pretty tablecloth, flowers, and a candle.

Carol Jackson lives alone. She works behind a counter in a department store all day. Her feet hurt when she gets home, and she's tired. Yet she has learned to make an occasion out of her dinner. She takes a bath, puts on a glamorous caftan, and sets a pretty place mat and napkin on her table with a candle and a single flower. She plays her favorite music on her stereo while she dines in good company—herself.

She has also learned the secret that if you don't have your problem foods in your house, chances are you won't eat them. That means shopping wisely.

∎ *Shop only after you have eaten, and always from a list.* We all react strongly to the sight of food when we are hungry. A hungry dieter with an empty basket in a supermarket is just asking for trouble. Cans and cartons of food seem to leap off the shelves into the shopping cart: Even if you do not buy your problem foods, the sight of them when you are hungry will linger in your mind, replaying the tape of deprivation for a long time afterward. If you go to the store with a full stomach and a complete list of the items needed for the coming week, you'll be able to shop quickly and efficiently.

▮ *Do not buy your problem foods.* No matter how careful your advance planning, you will probably find at least one aisle in the supermarket virtually impassable. There are some of us who can't get by sour cream; others who run aground in the cookie section, and still others who zero in on the mixed nuts like a magnet. Psychological studies have shown that the closer you are to a food item, the greater your desire for the food. So it is better to leave those temptations in the supermarket and eliminate the need to deal with them at home. Do not bring them into your home. Do not serve them. Later, when you've reprogrammed yourself into thin behavior, you will be able to confront these special problem foods and eat them within reason.

▮ *Reprogram your schedule.* Too often, we find ourselves eating something automatically because some event or emotion has set off an old eating association. After work we stop at the grocery store; we take the groceries home, and while putting them away, we have just a bite of this or a tiny sample of that. It is possible, however, to break that chain of events leading to automatic snacking by observing our own behavior. Pinpoint the specific events in the chain and find a spot to break the chain. You can break the chain that leads to after-work eating, for example, by not going to the food store after work. Instead, take a walk or a shower or a nap, or buy your food after dinner. If you do go to the store and find yourself pulling into the driveway with a big bag of food, break the chain there; leave the groceries in the car and carry them in after dinner, or send the kids out to get them and put them away. You will probably continue to hear those old tapes playing, trying to lead you into the familiar "chaining" process—"home at last; time for a little something"—but you can break that chain.

■ *Deal with family pitfalls.* The overweight person who has to shop for and serve food to the whole family has problems, as most of us well know. What do you do about the rest of the people for whom you prepare meals? We advise you to prepare Lean Line meals for the entire family because the Lean Line Program is a well-balanced, nutritious eating plan that is healthy for everyone. Members of your family who are not overweight need not be as careful as you about the amount of food they eat, but simply by eating the way you do, they will eliminate a lot of the sugars and fried foods that are not good for them.

Your family may want to help you lose weight by joining in on your One Month Lighter Program; but if they insist on different foods, let them take the responsibility of buying, preparing, serving, and cleaning up after eating those items. If family members can't get along without an item that's a problem for you, let them handle it themselves. If Junior takes charge of his own ice cream, you can think of it as *his* food. Even when you come across it in the freezer, you will be less tempted to eat it if you know that it doesn't belong to you. You have, in this manner, created what psychologists call distance between yourself and food.

Karen Wilson, a self-proclaimed earth mother, had maintained she would feel guilty if she made her preteen children take responsibility for their own food. After all, they had a right to have their meals created and prepared for them by a loving mother. We explained to her that what she would be doing for her family was the same thing she would be doing for herself. She would create healthy, independent human beings responsible for their own welfare. Karen confessed afterward that she probably was reluctant to let her kids take over their own meals because she was the chief consumer of some of the foods she had kept on hand "for the children." She stopped baking the weekly brownies she'd said her kids "couldn't live without"—but none of them even noticed.

▌*Choose your own basic food program.* Lean Line does not impose irrational rules about what you may and may not eat. Marjorie, who has become one of our lecturers, laughs about it now and tells every group what she did the hour before she came to her first Lean Line lecture: "I ate six bran muffins slathered with butter because I thought I was never going to eat them again. The suggested breakfast for the first week of the Lean Line Program was *bran muffins.*"

We suggest a basic food program—not a deprivation diet—and ask you to take responsibility for yourself. If you don't follow the One Month Lighter Program perfectly, it will not be a disaster, any more than it will be a disaster if you forget your behavior modification techniques from time to time. But if you choose to stick closely to the program for just four weeks, you will be delighted at the weight you will lose and the changes in your eating habits.

4. THE ONE MONTH LIGHTER PROGRAM

Who said that good things to eat have to be fattening? Remember what we said about food being a sensuous experience? Not only should your food taste good but it should look good, smell good, and feel good in your mouth—to say nothing about your digestive system. All it takes is a little creativity.

In the One Month Lighter Program, we've given you meal plans that are fast and easy to prepare for those times when you have little time. We've also given you gourmet recipes, which require slightly more preparation. All recipes, however, carefully take into account calories, nutrition, taste, and eye appeal, and conform one hundred percent to the official Lean Line Program.

It is of the utmost importance that you make your meals

as attractive as possible and thoroughly enjoy the food that you eat so that you will learn to be truly satisfied.

The program, as we have emphasized, involves choices. It allows for the widest variety in both the personality of the eater and the food to be eaten. Even if you follow the program from page 44 to page 164 exactly as we have laid it out, you will still be able to pick and choose a wide variety of dishes. The Lean Line Program is remarkably easy to follow because it offers you an opportunity to eat the foods you most enjoy and lose weight while doing so. Lolly hasn't given up her bagels and potato pancakes, and Toni hasn't denied herself lasagna and antipasto.

There are *six* basic food lists (see Chapter 9) from which you will be selecting your food intake for the day. These are the Protein, Vegetable, Bread, Milk, Fruit, Oil and Condiment lists. There are also two Bonus Lists, but items on them are not required.

One protein selection at each meal is a requirement. You may not like the one we selected for you at a particular meal. Feel free to substitute another protein from the same Protein List. There are four Protein Lists: A, B, C, and D. They vary in calories and the source of protein. Check the top of each list carefully for the correct portion of protein allotted at breakfast, lunch, and dinner. There are suggested limits per week for List C, the one that contains cheese and eggs, because of cholesterol content. We urge you to vary your protein selections for maximum weight loss, interest, and nutrition.

There are three vegetable lists: A, B, and C. Once again, you should check the top of each list for the correct amount for a meal. You should have at least one vegetable a day. List B contains vegetables higher in calories than the others, so selections from that list should be chosen only three times a week. The vegetables from List C may be used freely without weighing or measuring, but try to avoid stuffing yourself with them. You want to change old behaviors, and overeating is a fat behavior. Try to use fresh or frozen vegetables, but if you have to use canned, buy the no-salt-added ones if possible.

Bake or broil your meat, fish, or poultry on a rack. You may use a nonstick pan or a no-stick vegetable cooking spray so long as you carefully keep pouring off the fat as it comes out of the meat, fish, or poultry. Microwave cooking is acceptable. Do not pot-roast, stew, or sauté meat, fish, or poultry.

Women should have two bread selections daily and men and preteens, three. Everyone should have two milk selections daily.

Women should have two fruit selections daily, and men and preteens, three. A vitamin C fruit selection is required daily. Fruits should be weighed with pits, peel, or skin wherever applicable. Use fresh, frozen, or canned fruit packed in unsweetened juice or water. Juice is measured separately. Never use fruit that has added sugar. Fresh whole fruit is preferred.

There is a list of oils and condiments, from which you can choose three selections daily, and a list of free foods, from which you can select generously within reason. There are five sticks of gum daily, for example, or bouillon or seltzer.

There are also two Bonus Lists you can use if you have utilized all foods on the program and are still hungry. You can take 2 ounces from Protein List B, for example, or another item from the Bread or Fruit list.

Lean Line strongly recommends drinking at least four 8-oz glasses of water or seltzer a day, before, during, or after meals. It flushes out the body and helps fill you up. Coffee, tea, and club soda do not fall into this category. Club soda has a lot of salt and gas in it. Coffee and tea have caffeine, which stimulates appetite. That is why we recommend decaffeinated coffee in our program. Herbal teas with no caffeine are okay too.

We have given you a complete One Month Lighter Program. No, we have given you *two* complete One Month Lighter Programs—a plain and a gourmet program, with every meal listed for each. However, if you do not like a particular dish or snack, merely substitute the appropriate one chosen from one of the food lists in Chapter 9. For example, if you don't like salmon, substitute ham. If you don't want okra, substitute bamboo shoots or winter squash. If you read Chapter 9 before beginning the One Month Lighter Program we've designed for you, you will be more adept at making substitutions.

The emphasis at Lean Line is on choices. The one real restriction, if you want the One Month Lighter Program to really work for you, is to weigh and/or measure all foods. For this purpose you will need a set of measuring spoons and a measuring cup, and we recommend a small kitchen or postal scale. You should also have an accurate bathroom scale to weigh yourself.

The program is planned within the structure of a twenty-four-hour period. Breakfast by 10 A.M., lunch and dinner repeated at the same time each day, the eating day ending at midnight. Anything other than free foods should be counted toward the next day's allowance.

OK, you are ready to start.

Now, set a goal weight for yourself. Make it reasonable. It is better to take weight off slowly. After all, it took you a long time to put that weight on. On the One Month Lighter Program, the average loss is two to five pounds per week, depending upon metabolism, previous eating habits, and the starting weight. The chart on page 37, will give you your approximate desired weight for your height and build.

Weigh yourself only once a week and at the same time of the day. In between, stay off the scales; minor fluctuations in your weight, often because of fluid retention or loss, may cause you needless anxiety if you weigh yourself daily. You may also want to record your waist measurement and keep a weekly record of inches lost. And, of course, before begin-

TABLE 1. DESIRABLE WEIGHTS FOR MEN AND WOMEN 25 YEARS OF AGE AND OVER (WEIGHED WITH INDOOR CLOTHING)

WOMEN

HEIGHT (IN SHOES) FT. IN.	SMALL FRAME	MEDIUM FRAME	LARGE FRAME
4 10	92— 98	96—107	104—119
4 11	94—101	98—110	106—122
5 0	96—104	101—113	109—125
5 1	99—107	104—116	112—128
5 2	102—110	107—119	115—131
5 3	105—113	110—122	118—134
5 4	108—116	113—126	121—138
5 5	111—119	116—130	125—142
5 6	114—123	120—135	129—146
5 7	118—127	124—139	133—150
5 8	122—131	128—143	137—154
5 9	126—135	132—147	141—158
5 10	130—140	136—151	145—163
5 11	134—144	140—155	149—168
6 0	138—148	144—159	153—173

MEN

HEIGHT (IN SHOES) FT. IN.	SMALL FRAME	MEDIUM FRAME	LARGE FRAME
5 2	112—120	118—129	126—141
5 3	115—123	121—133	129—144
5 4	118—126	124—136	132—148
5 5	121—129	127—139	135—152
5 6	124—133	130—143	138—156
5 7	128—137	134—147	142—162
5 8	132—141	138—152	147—166
5 9	136—145	142—156	151—170
5 10	140—150	146—160	155—174
5 11	144—154	150—165	159—179
6 0	148—158	154—170	164—184
6 1	152—162	158—175	168—189
6 2	156—167	162—180	173—194
6 3	160—171	167—185	178—199
6 4	164—175	172—190	182—204

Statistical data from Metropolitan Life Insurance Co.

ning this or any other diet program, you should consult your doctor.

The One Month Lighter Program has been carefully designed to be safe, nutritious, and fun and to provide maximum success with minimum effort. Now, begin to be thin!

Before You Begin

Before beginning Week 1 of the One Month Lighter Program, please read the following.

▌ All recipes are for one serving unless otherwise indicated.

▌ All recipe portions are for women; men and preteens should check lists (beginning on page 168) for additional amounts.

▌ All calories given for each recipe are approximations.

▌ Measurements for beef, pork, poultry, and fish:
One 3-oz serving is equivalent to 1 slice approximately ½ in. thick, 3½ in. long, and 2 in. wide or 2 slices approximately ¼ in. thick and 3½ in. in length.

▌ Butter, margarine, mayonnaise, and other fats, unless specified as "imitation," are real.

▌ Unprocessed bran, which is used to add fiber to your diet, may be obtained in most supermarkets and health-food stores. Consider it optional if unattainable. It should be mixed with cereals when listed as a plain breakfast item.

▌ Large tossed salads may include any combination of vegetables from Vegetable List C (pages 173–74); variety is recommended.

▌ Coffee or tea may be used as desired; decaffeinated coffee and herbal tea are recommended because regular coffee and tea may stimulate appetite in some people. See Free Food List (page 182) for other beverages.

▌ In menu plans and recipes, one egg is a medium-sized egg.

▌ In menu plans, any citrus fruit (see pages 177–78) may be substituted for 8 oz (½ medium) grapefruit.

▌ You must eat all the food on the meal plan each day. For

example, you are required to have three oil and condiment Selections each day. If you do not wish to put the specified low-calorie dressing on your salad, then you must substitute 1 oil and condiment selection (see page 179) because you need oil in your diet.

■ We recommend you use caution, but as far as calories and blood sugar levels are concerned, you may use as much sugar substitute each day as you wish with the exception of aspartame. You should not exceed four packets of aspartame per day.

■ Our menu plans provide a lot of flexibility. You may eat plain one day and gourmet the next. Or you may switch Monday's meals with Thursday's. You may substitute items from the same lists in Chapter 9 or mix and match among the lists, but you should not eat a *gourmet* breakfast and a *plain* lunch until you have learned to formulate your own diet plan. In the One Month Lighter Program we designed for you, everything has been carefully balanced according to a *plain meal day* or a *gourmet meal day*.

Before making any substitutions—and you certainly can make them in the One Month Lighter Program we designed for you—read Chapter 9.

5. CHOOSE
TO LOSE—
WEEK 1

Why do you want to be thin?

Each of us has our own personal reason. We also have our schedules, obligations, and personality characteristics.

Tara, for example, is the very epitome of the smart, dynamic, successful career woman. As a child, she was a tomboy, always competing with her four brothers. After receiving her master's degree in business, she was on a fast track as a financial consultant. She had little time to learn to cook. She was always ten to fifteen pounds overweight but never did anything about it until she heard two secretaries talking in the ladies' room one day: "Tara would be pretty if she wasn't so heavy." That remark made her decide finally to do something about her excess weight.

"I always research everything I do, and I researched a diet

program," Tara said. "I asked people which ones worked for them and how long they were able to keep the weight off. I talked it over with some medical friends to see which diets they thought were well balanced. They recommended the Lean Line Program. I attended an introductory class and told the lecturer that I didn't have more time to fuss with my meals than before I began the program. She told me I didn't have to and I didn't. I actually found it easier to plan and fix my meals, and I can keep to the program even when I travel for business."

Tara lost twelve pounds. It has been a little more than a year that she's maintained her weight, but knowing Tara, we are sure she is going to keep it off permanently.

Louann, on the other hand, only wanted to be a wife and mother. She literally had been on a "crash" diet when she came to Lean Line.

"My husband, Jim, and I always wanted a big family. Each time I had a baby, I gained weight. With my last daughter, my weight blossomed from one hundred and forty-one pounds to one hundred and eighty-two, and after she was born, I still weighed one hundred and seventy-eight pounds, and I'm five feet five. I had vowed to lose weight and I had tried a diet for a week or so, and then I went back to my old fat habits.

"Three weeks after the birth of our last baby, my husband was taking me to the supermarket when another driver crashed into us. I wasn't hurt but Jim was almost killed.

"When it was touch-and-go at the hospital and it looked like I might lose Jim, I lost weight. Between taking care of the new baby and two toddlers and running back and forth to the hospital, never knowing when that awful phone call would come, I had no appetite. But when he came home, he needed constant care. I couldn't leave the house, and with three small children, I felt trapped. I ate and ate from boredom, relief, and anxiety all mixed together. I reached one hundred and ninety pounds.

"Jim was able to return to work a year after the accident, and I decided I had to do something about the way I looked. My neighbor suggested Lean Line.

"I love to cook as well as eat, but, of course, with three small kids, I didn't have too much time. I expected the diet to be a sort of punishment that I had to go through. Instead, I found I could still eat all my favorites—even apple pie and ice cream—and I learned a lot of new recipes and cooking shortcuts. I lost fifty-seven pounds in nine months, and I've never had more energy.

"Jim and I went on our first vacation alone in six years. He kept telling me I looked like a new woman, and when we stood in front of the motel desk clerk waiting to check in, Jim looked at me and said, 'What did you say your name was, Miss?' We still laugh about it, but, honestly, I really do feel like a new and very lucky person."

Cindy is another Lean Liner who became a new woman. She had let herself become fat and frowsy and boring. When she lost thirty pounds, she fixed her hair in a new style, bought new clothes, and for the first time in years became interested in sex. Unfortunately for her husband, not with him. She divorced him, remarried, and sends us glowing letters periodically about all the fun she is having as a "thin person."

Why do you want to be thin? Is it because your job depends on it? Is it because your lover wants you to be thin? What force is pulling you to be thin? If you are not sure, or if the force is not generated from within yourself, then forget about being thin. You'll never make it in a thin world.

The need to be thin must come from within you; the need to be thin must be greater than all the temptations that lead you to overeat. Many people say that in order to be thin, you must have *willpower*. We disagree. You must have *want power*. You must want to be thin because you want to be thin, because you enjoy the feeling of achievement when you lose weight. You must want to be thin because being thin can release the creative forces that ultimately will make you the complete human being you were meant to be.

Unless *you* have this *want power,* no book, no person, no diet, can make a difference.

The following One Month Lighter Program can work for you. However, it is not romantic. It won't grab you and beat you into submission. It requires your commitment. A month is not a long time. It is achievable. Try it.

(Note: an asterisk after a menu suggestion indicates that the recipe follows.)

DAY 1 PLAIN

Breakfast

8 oz (½ medium) grapefruit

1 egg (not to exceed 5 per week) or *2 oz (¼ cup) low-fat cottage cheese* or *1 oz (1 slice) hard cheese (not to exceed 4 oz per week)* or *1 oz (¼ cup) wheat germ*

4 oz (½ cup) cooked cereal or *¾ oz (¾ cup) dry cereal*

2 tablespoons unprocessed bran

8 oz (1 cup) skim milk

Lunch

Large tossed salad

4 teaspoons low-calorie salad dressing

4 oz cooked white turkey meat

Dinner

Large tossed salad

4 teaspoons low-calorie salad dressing

3 oz roast beef

4 oz (½ cup) cooked squash

Add to or between meals 1 Bread Selection (see page 175), 1 Milk Selection (see page 176), and 1 Fruit Selection (see pages 177–78).

DAY 1 GOURMET

Breakfast

8 oz (½ medium) grapefruit

1 soft-boiled egg

Lunch

* Cottage Tuna Salad Open-faced Sandwich

* Tomato Surprise

8 oz (1 cup) skim milk

Dinner

6 oz roasted white turkey meat

* Mushroom Gravy

3 oz (⅓ cup) cooked whole-grain rice

4 oz (½ cup) whole-kernel corn

* Steamed Broccoli Italiano

4 oz (½ cup) grapes

Add to or between meals 1 Milk Selection (see page 176).

DAY 1 GOURMET
RECIPES

▮ COTTAGE TUNA SALAD OPEN-FACED SANDWICH ▮
145 calories

2 oz (¼ cup) low-fat cottage cheese
1 oz (⅛ cup) water-packed tuna
Onion powder to taste
1 oz (1 slice) pumpernickel bread

Mix together cottage cheese, tuna, and onion powder. Spread mixture on bread.

COUNTS AS: 1 Lunch Protein List B
1 Bread Selection

▮ TOMATO SURPRISE ▮
55 calories

4 oz (1 small) tomato
½ stalk celery, finely chopped
2 teaspoons imitation mayonnaise

Carefully scoop out center of tomato and reserve shell. Place chopped celery and tomato pulp in bowl, and mix well with mayonnaise. Spoon back into tomato shell.

COUNTS AS: 1 Oil and Condiment Selection
1 Vegetable List C

▌ STEAMED BROCCOLI ITALIANO ▌
165 calories

1 10-oz package fresh or frozen broccoli
4 tablespoons wine vinegar
2 teaspoons vegetable oil
⅛ teaspoon dried oregano
⅛ teaspoon dried basil
⅛ teaspoon grated Parmesan cheese
Garlic powder and black pepper to taste
Salt to taste (optional)

Cook broccoli according to package directions and drain well. Combine remaining ingredients and toss with broccoli. Serve hot.

COUNTS AS: 2 Oil and Condiment Selections

▌ MUSHROOM GRAVY ▌
20 calories

1 small can (⅓ cup) water-packed, sliced mushrooms, undrained, or ⅓ cup fresh mushrooms with water to cover
1 packet chicken bouillon powder, undissolved

Blend mushrooms with liquid in blender for 10 seconds. Add bouillon and continue blending for additional 5 seconds. Pour mixture into 1-quart saucepan and heat over medium heat until hot.

COUNTS AS: Free Food

DAY 2 PLAIN

Breakfast

8 oz (½ medium) grapefruit

1 egg or 2 oz (¼ cup) low-fat cottage cheese

4 oz (½ cup) cooked cereal or ¾ oz (¾ cup)
dry cereal

2 tablespoons unprocessed bran

8 oz (1 cup) skim milk

Lunch

Large tossed salad

4 teaspoons low-calorie salad dressing

4 oz (½ cup) water-packed tuna

1 oz (½ large) whole-wheat pita bread

2 teaspoons imitation mayonnaise

Sprouts (as desired)

Dinner

Large tossed salad

4 teaspoons low-calorie salad dressing

4–6 oz cooked white turkey meat

4 oz (½ medium) tomato

4 oz (½ cup) cooked sliced carrots

Add to or between meals 1 Milk Selection (see
page 176) and 1 Fruit Selection (see pages
177–78).

DAY 2 GOURMET

Breakfast

8 oz (½ medium) grapefruit

1 oz (¼ cup) wheat germ

¾ oz (⅔ cup) shredded wheat

2 tablespoons unprocessed bran

8 oz (1 cup) skim milk

Lunch

Large tossed salad

4 teaspoons low-calorie salad dressing

* Open-Faced Shrimp Sandwich

Dinner

Large tossed salad

4 teaspoons low-calorie salad dressing

* Polynesian Chicken

Add to or between meals 1 Milk Selection (see page 176).

DAY 2 GOURMET
RECIPES

❙ OPEN-FACED SHRIMP SANDWICH ❙
275 calories

2 oz (¼ cup) cooked shrimp
1 oz (½ medium) English muffin, toasted lightly and buttered
1 teaspoon butter
1 oz (1 thin slice) natural cheddar cheese, grated

Place shrimp on muffin. Top with grated cheese and broil until cheese melts.

COUNTS AS: 1 Lunch Protein combined Lists B and C
1 Bread Selection
1 Oil and Condiment Selection

❙ POLYNESIAN CHICKEN ❙
355 calories

8 oz chicken cutlets (will cook down to 6 oz)
6 oz (¾ cup) tomato juice
1 tablespoon soy sauce
3 oz (1 medium) green pepper, chopped
2 oz (¼ cup) chopped onions
½ stalk celery, finely chopped
4 oz (½ cup) canned unsweetened crushed pineapple, undrained

Broil chicken on rack. Let cool and cut into chunks. In saucepan, combine tomato juice, soy sauce, pepper, onions, celery, and pineapple with juice. Cook uncovered over low heat. When sauce thickens, add chicken, stir, and serve. Entire dish takes about a half hour to cook.

COUNTS AS: 1 Dinner Protein List B
               ½ Vegetable List A Selection
               1 Fruit Selection
               Daily soy sauce from Free Food List

DAY 3 PLAIN

Breakfast

8 oz (½ medium) grapefruit

1 soft-boiled egg

4 oz (½ cup) cooked farina

2 tablespoons unprocessed bran

8 oz (1 cup) skim milk

Lunch

Large tossed salad

4 teaspoons low-calorie salad dressing

2 oz cooked hamburger

Dinner

Large tossed salad

4 teaspoons low-calorie salad dressing

6 oz broiled filet of sole

3 oz (⅓ cup) cooked brown rice

1 teaspoon butter

4 oz (½ cup) cooked sliced beets

Add to or between meals 1 Milk Selection (see page 176) and 1 Fruit Selection (see pages 177–78).

DAY 3 GOURMET

Breakfast

8 oz (½ medium) grapefruit

1 soft-boiled egg

4 oz (½ cup) cooked farina

2 tablespoons unprocessed bran

8 oz (1 cup) skim milk

Lunch

Large tossed salad

4 teaspoons low-calorie salad dressing

* Vegetarian Delight

1 oz (¾ medium) bran muffin

1 teaspoon butter

Dinner

Large tossed salad

4 teaspoons low-calorie salad dressing

* Turkey Ratatouille

DAY 3 GOURMET
RECIPES

∎ VEGETARIAN DELIGHT ∎
335 calories

4 oz (½ cup) low-fat plain yogurt
Artificial sweetener (to equal the sweetness of 4 teaspoons sugar)
¼ teaspoon vanilla extract
4 oz (½ cup) mixed fresh fruits (berries, apples, etc.)
1 oz (¼ cup) wheat germ
½ oz (1 tablespoon) chopped mixed nuts

Place yogurt in serving dish. Add artificial sweetener and vanilla, and mix well. Add fruit and mix. Top with wheat germ and nuts.

COUNTS AS: 1 Lunch Protein List D
1 Fruit Selection
1 Milk Selection
1 Oil Selection

∎ TURKEY RATATOUILLE ∎
(4 servings) 325 calories per serving

12 oz (1½ cups) tomato juice
Sprinkling of onion flakes
1 clove garlic, minced
1 tablespoon chopped, fresh or dried, parsley
1 bay leaf
24 oz (3 cups) diced cooked white turkey meat
16 oz (2 cups) cooked diced and peeled eggplant
16 oz (3 cups) cooked diced zucchini

Combine tomato juice, onion flakes, garlic, parsley, and bay leaf. Toss lightly with turkey and vegetables until blended well. Bake, uncovered, at 325° for 15 minutes. Remove bay leaf and serve.

EACH SERVING COUNTS AS: 1 Dinner Protein List B
3 oz tomato juice from Free Food List
1 Vegetable List C

DAY 4 PLAIN

Breakfast

8 oz (½ medium) grapefruit
1 oz (¼ cup) wheat germ
¾ oz (⅔ cup) shredded wheat
2 tablespoons unprocessed bran
8 oz (1 cup) skim milk

Lunch

Large tossed salad

4 teaspoons low-calorie salad dressing

4 oz (½ cup) low-fat cottage cheese

Dinner

Large tossed salad

4 teaspoons low-calorie salad dressing

3 oz broiled lean beef

4 oz (½ medium) baked potato with

4 teaspoons sour cream

Add to or between meals 1 Bread Selection (see page 175), 1 Milk Selection (see page 176), and 1 Fruit Selection (see pages 177–78).

DAY 4 GOURMET

Breakfast

8 oz (½ medium) grapefruit

* Bread Custard Pudding

Lunch

Large tossed salad

4 teaspoons low-calorie salad dressing

* Noontime Fruit Salad

Dinner

Large tossed salad

4 teaspoons low-calorie salad dressing

---

* Shrimp Chow Mein

---

3 oz (⅓ cup) cooked brown rice with

---

1 teaspoon butter

Add to or between meals 1 Milk Selection (see page 176).

DAY 4 GOURMET RECIPES

▌ BREAD CUSTARD PUDDING ▌
230 calories

---

1 oz (1 slice) bread, cubed

---

1 egg

Artificial sweetener (to equal sweetness of 6 teaspoons sugar)

---

1 teaspoon vanilla extract

---

2 tablespoons unprocessed bran

---

8 oz (1 cup) skim milk

Ground cinnamon and nutmeg to taste

Place bread in baking dish. In separate dish, combine egg, sweetener, vanilla, and bran; then blend in milk. Pour over bread cubes, and sprinkle with cinnamon and nutmeg. Set baking dish in pan of warm water and place in oven. Bake uncovered at 350° for 1 hour. Let cool and enjoy.

COUNTS AS: 1 Breakfast Protein List C *or* 1 Bonus List A Selection
1 Bread Selection
1 Milk Selection

▮ NOONTIME FRUIT SALAD ▮
(2 servings) 75 calories per serving

1 box sugar-free lemon or lime gelatin
1½ oz (½ cup) grated cabbage
8 oz (1 cup) low-fat cottage cheese
8 oz (1 cup) canned unsweetened crushed pine-apple, drained
2 oz (¼ cup) diced green pepper

Prepare gelatin according to package directions. When practically set, add remaining ingredients. Refrigerate until firm.

EACH SERVING COUNTS AS: 1 Lunch Protein List C
1 Fruit Selection

▮ SHRIMP CHOW MEIN ▮
300 calories

1 packet onion bouillon powder or 1 bouillon cube
8 oz (1 cup) hot water
½ teaspoon garlic powder
3 oz (1 medium) green pepper, cut into strips
2 small celery stalks, sliced
2 oz (¼ cup) onions, cut into strips
6 oz (2 cups) shredded raw cabbage
2 oz (¼ cup) whole snow peas
6 oz (¾ cup) cooked shrimp
4 oz (½ cup) bean sprouts
2 oz (¼ cup) canned or fresh sliced mushrooms
Salt and pepper to taste

In saucepan or wok, dissolve bouillon in hot water with garlic powder. Add green pepper, celery, onion, cabbage, and snow peas, and cook until barely tender. Add remaining ingredients, and simmer uncovered briefly until flavors blend.

COUNTS AS: 1 Dinner Protein List B
1 Vegetable List A Selection

DAY 5 PLAIN

Breakfast

8 oz (½ medium) grapefruit
1 hard-boiled egg
¾ oz (1½ cup) puffed rice
2 tablespoons unprocessed bran
8 oz (1 cup) skim milk

Lunch

Large tossed salad
4 teaspoons low-calorie salad dressing
2–4 oz cooked white turkey meat
1 oz (1 slice) rye bread
1 teaspoon mayonnaise

Dinner

Large tossed salad
4 teaspoons low-calorie salad dressing
4–6 oz broiled trout
4 oz (½ cup) brussels sprouts

Add to or between meals 1 Milk Selection (see page 176), and 1 Fruit Selection (see pages 177–78).

DAY 5 GOURMET

Breakfast

4 oz (½ cup) grapefruit sections

* High Fiber Loaf

4 oz (½ cup) skim milk

Lunch

Large tossed salad

4 teaspoons low-calorie salad dressing

* Easy Peas and Macaroni

Dinner

Large tossed salad

4 teaspoons low-calorie salad dressing

* Zucchini Lasagna made with

Lean Line Tomato Sauce

Add to or between meals 1 Milk Selection (see page 176) and 1 Fruit Selection (see pages 177–78).

DAY 5 GOURMET
RECIPES

∎ HIGH FIBER LOAF ∎
(4 servings) 200 calories per serving

2 oz (1 cup) 100% bran cereal
½ cup unprocessed bran
2 packets sugar-free chocolate-flavor mix
8 oz (1 cup) orange juice
4 eggs
½ teaspoon ground cloves
½ teaspoon ground allspice
½ teaspoon grated orange peel
Ground cinnamon, vanilla extract, and artificial sweetener to taste
1½ teaspoons baking powder

Soak bran cereal, unprocessed bran, and cocoa mix in orange juice until completely absorbed. Add remaining ingredients and beat for 3 minutes at medium speed with hand mixer. Turn out into loaf pan coated with no-stick cooking vegetable spray, and bake at 350° for 20 minutes.

EACH SERVING COUNTS AS: 1 Breakfast Protein List C
¾ Bread Selection
¼ Fruit Selection
½ Milk Selection

▮ EASY PEAS AND MACARONI ▮
250 calories

4 oz (½ cup) green peas
3 oz (⅓ cup) cooked enriched elbow macaroni or 3 oz (⅓ cup) cooked brown rice
4 oz (½ cup) home-style meatless oil-free tomato sauce
3 oz (1 medium) cooked green pepper, diced
Onion salt to taste

Mix together all ingredients and heat in saucepan until warm.

COUNTS AS: 1 Dinner Protein List D
1 Vegetable List A Selection
1 Bread Selection

▮ ZUCCHINI LASAGNA ▮
(2 servings) 430 calories per serving

4 teaspoons imitation margarine
2 oz (¼ cup) chopped onions
8 oz (1 cup) Lean Line Tomato Sauce (see page 197)
⅛ teaspoon salt
¼ teaspoon dried oregano
6 oz (about 8 noodles) cooked enriched lasagna noodles
10 oz (2 cups) cooked sliced zucchini
5 oz part-skim mozzarella cheese, sliced
1 oz (2 tablespoons) grated Parmesan cheese

Melt margarine in skillet. Add onions and sauté until limp. Add tomato sauce, salt, and oregano. Cover and simmer for 30 minutes, stirring occasionally. In baking dish, layer half the noodles, top with half the zucchini, half the tomato sauce, and half the mozzarella. Repeat. Top with Parmesan cheese. Bake uncovered at 375 ° for 20–25 minutes.

COUNTS AS: 1 Dinner Protein List C
¼ Vegetable List A Selection
1 Bread Selection
1 Oil and Condiment Selection
Daily tomato juice from Free Food List

DAY 6 PLAIN

Breakfast

8 oz (½ medium) grapefruit
1 egg scrambled with 2 tablespoons unprocessed bran
1 oz (1 slice) whole-wheat toast
1 teaspoon butter
8 oz (1 cup) skim milk

Lunch

Large tossed salad
4 teaspoons low-calorie salad dressing
2 oz lean roast beef
8 oz (1 cup) fresh strawberries

Dinner

Large tossed salad
4 teaspoons low-calorie salad dressing

4-6 oz broiled halibut

4 oz (½ cup) peas

Add to or between meals 1 Bread Selection (see page 175) and 1 Milk Selection (see page 176).

DAY 6 GOURMET

Breakfast

8 oz (½ medium) grapefruit

* 2 Bran Muffins

8 oz (1 cup) skim milk

Lunch

Large tossed salad

4 teaspoons low-calorie salad dressing

* Broccoli Supreme

Dinner

Large tossed salad

4 teaspoons low-calorie salad dressing

* Shrimp Creole

Add to or between meals ½ Milk Selection (see page 176) and 1 Fruit Selection (see pages 177-78).

DAY 6 GOURMET
RECIPES

▮ BRAN MUFFINS ▮
(6 muffins, 3 servings)
180 calories per serving

3 oz (1½ cups) 100% bran cereal
Artificial sweetener (to equal sweetness of 6 teaspoons sugar)
2 teaspoons baking powder
6 tablespoons unprocessed bran
3 eggs
3 teaspoons vanilla extract
3 oz (⅓ cup) water

Combine cereal, sweetener, baking powder, and bran. Add eggs, vanilla, and water. Mix thoroughly, and let stand for 5 minutes. Spoon into nonstick muffin tins or muffin tins coated with nostick vegetable cooking spray. Bake at 350° for 25 minutes, or until golden brown.

2 MUFFINS COUNT AS: 1 Breakfast Protein List C
1 Bread Selection

▮ BROCCOLI SUPREME ▮
318 calories

1 10-oz package frozen broccoli or 1⅓ cups fresh broccoli
4 oz (½ cup) buttermilk
2 oz (2 slices) cheddar cheese
Salt and pepper to taste

Cook broccoli according to package directions and set aside. Place buttermilk and cheese in saucepan and simmer over medium heat for 5 minutes. Stir constantly to avoid scorching. Season with salt and pepper. Place broccoli on serving dish and pour cheese sauce over it.

COUNTS AS: 1 Lunch Protein List C
$\qquad$ ½ Milk Selection

▮ SHRIMP CREOLE ▮
350 calories

8 oz (1 cup) tomato juice
2 teaspoons imitation margarine
1 oz (2 tablespoons) minced onions
1 oz (2 tablespoons) chopped celery
1 oz (2 tablespoons) chopped green pepper
Salt and pepper to taste
6 oz (¾ cup) cooked peeled shrimp
3 oz (⅓ cup) cooked enriched white rice

In saucepan, over medium heat, reduce tomato juice by almost half. In skillet, heat margarine and brown onions, celery, and green pepper in it. Add to tomato juice in saucepan and simmer uncovered for 15 minutes. Add shrimp and heat. Serve over cooked rice.

COUNTS AS: 1 Dinner Protein List B
$\qquad$ ¼ Vegetable List A Selection
$\qquad$ 1 Bread Selection
$\qquad$ 1 Oil and Condiment Selection
$\qquad$ Daily tomato juice from Free Food List

DAY 7 PLAIN

Breakfast

8 oz (½ medium) grapefruit

2 oz (¼ cup) low-fat cottage cheese

¾ oz (½ cup) bran flakes

2 tablespoons unprocessed bran

8 oz (1 cup) skim milk

Lunch

Large tossed salad

4 teaspoons low-calorie salad dressing

2–4 oz cooked white turkey meat

Dinner

Large tossed salad

4 teaspoons low-calorie salad dressing

3 oz broiled flank steak

4 oz (½ medium) baked potato with

4 teaspoons sour cream

Add to or between meals 1 Bread Selection (see page 175), 1 Milk Selection (see page 176), and 1 Fruit Selection (see pages 177–78).

DAY 7 GOURMET

Breakfast

* Connie's Apple Chews

Lunch

8 oz (½ medium) grapefruit

Large tossed salad

4 teaspoons low-calorie salad dressing

2 oz lean roast beef

Dinner

Large tossed salad

4 teaspoons low-calorie salad dressing

* Chicken and Roasted Peppers

4 oz (½ cup) mashed butternut squash with

1 teaspoon butter

Add to or between meals 1 Bread Selection (see page 175) and 1 Milk Selection (see page 176).

DAY 7 GOURMET
RECIPES

▮ CONNIE'S APPLE CHEWS ▮

(2 servings) 333 calories per serving

2 4-oz apples (medium, 2½ in. diameter), unpeeled and sliced into chunks
4 oz (½ cup) low-fat plain yogurt
⅓ cup nonfat dry milk
1½ oz (1½ cups) mixed cereals (100% bran, wheat flakes, oatmeal)
2 tablespoons unprocessed bran
2 beaten eggs
1 tablespoon vanilla extract
1 tablespoon ground cinnamon (or to taste)
Artificial sweetener (to equal sweetness of 4 teaspoons sugar)

Preheat oven to 500°. Mix together all ingredients in pie plate. Reduce oven to 400° and bake for 20–25 minutes.

EACH SERVING COUNTS AS: 1 Breakfast Protein List C Selection
1 Bread Selection
1 Fruit Selection
1 Milk Selection
Daily vanilla extract from Free Food List

▌ CHICKEN AND ROASTED PEPPERS ▐
405 calories

1 8-oz jar (1 cup) water-packed roasted red peppers, drained
8 oz (1 cup) tomato juice
1 teaspoon freshly squeezed lemon juice
Salt, pepper, and oregano to taste
8 oz boneless chicken breast (will cook down to 6 oz)

Mix together roasted peppers, tomato juice, lemon juice, salt, pepper, and oregano. Add chicken and marinate for about 4 hours. Reserve marinade. Bake chicken at 350° on rack. Pour warmed marinade over cooked chicken and serve.

COUNTS AS: 1 Dinner Protein List B
          Daily tomato juice from Free Food List

6. STRESS, THE GREAT DIET DESTROYER— WEEK 2

Sandra Klepper was going through a divorce. Every time her lawyer called, she could hardly talk to him because her mouth was full. She was easing her pain temporarily with food—but only temporarily, because when she looked in the mirror, she hated what she saw and she could understand, almost, why her husband had an affair with a woman at the office.

Jane Whitney's son was awaiting word from the only college he wished to attend. It was her job to open the mail and call him at school if the acceptance came. The tension in the house was all-consuming; each day just about noon, when the mailman was expected, Jane would start eating her lunch. It was a long, long lunch.

Lisa Brownstern had a high-pressured advertising job.

When she was under pressure—as she often was—she would go to the candy or soda machine and fill her mouth while she thought about the next layout.

How do you handle stress? If you are reading this book and you're like the rest of us, you probably ease tension by putting something in your mouth.

Stress exists in everyday life. Whenever you are in a situation where you feel tense, what happens? Your stomach tightens up, you have difficulty concentrating or sleeping. Sticking to a diet program adds still more stress to your life. But you can either decide it's hopeless or learn to relieve stress related to dieting and at the same time relieve other stresses in your life. Like eating properly, it is a matter of learning new behaviors.

Some of the stress involved in dieting comes from unrealistic expectations. You usually begin a diet by saying, "I have to lose weight," and then you tack on a time limit to add to the burden. If you believe that you have to lose ten pounds in two weeks, you are placing yourself in a stressful situation. What happens at the end of the first week if you've only lost three pounds? You are suddenly faced with losing seven pounds the next week.

You may say, "The heck with it," and lose control of your eating, a phenomenon called the binge.

"Binge" is the word that signals the beginning of the end for most dieters. It has absolutely nothing to do with hunger, which is a physiological drive for food. It has to do with appetite, which has to do with the desire to eat and may be based purely on psychological or environmental reasons, such as boredom or because everyone else is doing it. A binge is caused by an uncontrollable appetite or craving. It takes place when one bite is too much and the whole cake isn't enough.

Every dieter has encountered the binge. Lolly still can't take just one chocolate from a box of candy. A binge brings with it a feeling of despair and helplessness. How many times have you sat gorging yourself with cookies and asking yourself the question, "Why am I doing this to myself?"

Still, you were unable to stop. One binge lays the foundation for another. It is an unending cycle of overeating followed by guilt and yet another bout of eating. You can learn to break it and be free of binges.

If you keep a Food and Emotions Chart (there is a sample on page 74), you will see a binge pattern emerge. For each and every binge, you will probably find an emotional stress was present. It may have been because a repairman was late. It could just be the result of a broken fingernail. It may even be the stress caused by a happy, emotional event. We have learned over the years that whenever we are under stress, food offers a release—a temporary one at best. Eating to relieve tension has become a habit.

By keeping a diary, not just of what you eat but of how you feel at the time you eat, you will begin to recognize things that trigger a binge. Perhaps you will see yourself eating when there is nothing else to do or when you are overtired or whenever you eat at your mother's. Once you begin to see when you are vulnerable, you can begin to build defenses against those times.

Learn from experience how to stop yourself. You're probably saying, "I never stop myself." You do! How else could you begin again a weight-reduction program? Perhaps you talked yourself in and out of finishing off the pie and the half gallon of ice cream. Perhaps instead of finishing that box of candy, you removed yourself from temptation and went outside and did some gardening or found an interesting book to read. Try to recall your past successes in avoiding binges when you were tempted.

Once you have become aware, do something! Look at your watch, for example, and put off taking that first bite for ten minutes. In the refrigerator have an emergency kit of foods you can nibble on freely. Keep a picture of your old fat self taped to the refrigerator—take a good look. Do you still

FOOD AND EMOTIONS CHART

Record everything you eat for breakfast, lunch, and dinner, and circle it. Summarize your BASIC ID at each meal for later analysis.

BASIC ID	MONDAY	TUESDAY	WEDNESDAY	THURSDAY	FRIDAY	SATURDAY	SUNDAY
BEHAVIOR What are you doing when?	BREAKFAST	BREAKFAST	BREAKFAST	BREAKFAST	BREAKFAST	BREAKFAST	BREAKFAST
AFFECT Describe your emotions							
SENSATION Which senses, if any, are stimulated?	LUNCH	LUNCH	LUNCH	LUNCH	LUNCH	LUNCH	LUNCH
IMAGERY What are your mental pictures at this time?							
COGNITION What do you believe is going on?	DINNER	DINNER	DINNER	DINNER	DINNER	DINNER	DINNER
INTERPERSONAL What's happening with your relationships?							
DIET Any food problems?	SNACKS	SNACKS	SNACKS	SNACKS	SNACKS	SNACKS	SNACKS

want to eat? If worse comes to worse, you can always go to bed and pull the covers up over your head. Take some action! All the food in the world is not going to make you feel good about yourself. Getting your eating under control will!

Here are some techniques that we have found help reduce stress before it turns into fat.

- *Rest.* While dieting, make sure that you get plenty of rest. Exhaustion often mimics hunger. Many times you think you are hungry when, in reality, that sensation is really fatigue. If you are not sure whether you are hungry or tired, take ten minutes to sit down, put your feet up, and close your eyes. You can use a kitchen timer. By the end of this break, you will probably feel refreshed, and the urge to eat will have passed.
- *Be on guard.* Stress is imposed on us by other people—a boss, a spouse, children—because of the demands they make on us. Become assertive with others. Assertiveness simply means asking for what *you* want and *getting it.* How many times have you agreed to do something when you didn't have time or didn't want to? Learn to say no and mean it! By trying to live up to the expectations of others, you place an added burden on your own life. How many times have you gone off your diet at someone's urging? We call such diet destroyers friendly enemies. Sometimes it's even a spouse, who sees the person he or she loves "melting away" and feels insecure. Sometimes it's jealousy.

  Judy Lane, for example, had a witchy neighbor, Ann, who was always needling her. Judy had lost forty pounds over the summer and really looked good in her shorts. Ann, however, talked about everything else except Judy's new, svelte figure. Finally, Judy could stand it no longer and said, "Ann, aren't you going to say anything about my new figure?"

  Ann said, "Oh, I didn't notice."

Judy's retort was, "That's funny, your husband did!"

That response not only tickled Judy, it was an example of her new assertiveness that reduced the stress she used to feel when neighbor Ann would act unsupportively.

▌ *Take time out for yourself.* Plan a time each day that is just for you. Do exactly what you want to do, even if that something is just staring at the wall. Don't let anyone or anything interfere with *your time.*

▌ *Do what you have always wanted to do.* Can you think of five things you like to do that don't involve eating? Are there things you want to do and have never tried? Why can't you begin now?

This week take a chance! Try something new!

DAY 8 PLAIN

Breakfast

8 oz (½ medium) grapefruit

2 oz (¼ cup) low-fat cottage cheese

4 oz (½ cup) cooked farina

2 tablespoons unprocessed bran

8 oz (1 cup) skim milk

Lunch

Large tossed salad

4 tablespoons low-calorie salad dressing

2–4 oz (¼–½ cup) cooked shrimp

8 oz (1 cup) fresh strawberries with

4 tablespoons sour cream

Dinner

Large tossed salad
4 teaspoons low-calorie salad dressing
3 oz liver with
4 oz (½ cup) onions, fried in pan coated with no-stick vegetable cooking spray
Add to or between meals 1 Bread Selection (see page 175) and 1 Milk Selection (see page 176).

DAY 8 GOURMET

Breakfast

8 oz (½ medium) grapefruit
*Jonathan's Omelette
1 oz (¾ medium) bran muffin
8 oz (1 cup) skim milk

Lunch

*Spinach Salad
2 tablespoons unprocessed bran

Dinner

Large tossed salad
*Breaded Chicken Cutlets
Add to or between meals 1 Milk Selection (see page 176) and 1 Fruit Selection (see pages 177–78).

DAY 8 GOURMET
RECIPES

▮ JONATHAN'S OMELETTE ▮
120 calories

1 egg, beaten
1 oz (2 tablespoons) chopped onions
1½ oz (½ small) green pepper, chopped
2 oz (¼ cup) sliced fresh mushrooms
1 oz (2 tablespoons) home-style meatless oil-free tomato sauce

Cook egg, onions, pepper, and mushrooms in uncovered nonstick skillet or skillet coated with no-stick vegetable cooking spray. Arrange on plate. Top with tomato sauce.

COUNTS AS: 1 Breakfast Protein List C
½ Vegetable List A Selection

▌ SPINACH SALAD ▐
390 calories

3 oz (2 cups) fresh spinach, rinsed thoroughly and chopped
8 oz (1 cup) sliced fresh mushrooms
2 oz (¼ cup) chopped onions
1 tablespoon wine vinegar
1 teaspoon vegetable oil
½ teaspoon salt
½ teaspoon pepper
Artificial sweetener (to equal sweetness of 2 teaspoons sugar)
1 strip bacon, cooked until crisp, then crumbled
1 tablespoon lemon juice
2 hard-boiled eggs, diced or sliced

Combine all ingredients and serve.

COUNT AS: 1 Lunch Protein List C
½ Vegetable List A Selection
2 Oil and Condiment Selections

▌ BREADED CHICKEN CUTLETS ▐
395 calories

8 oz chicken or veal cutlets (will cook down to 6 oz)
4 teaspoons low-calorie clear French salad dressing
¾ oz (¾ cup) cornflakes, crushed

Marinate cutlets in salad dressing for several hours. Roll in corn-flakes. Bake on rack at 350° for 45 minutes. Delicious.

COUNTS AS: 1 Dinner Protein List B
1 Bread Selection
1 Oil and Condiment Selection

DAY 9 PLAIN

Breakfast

8 oz (½ medium) grapefruit

1 egg scrambled without butter or margarine

¾ oz (⅔ cup) shredded wheat

2 tablespoons unprocessed bran

8 oz (1 cup) skim milk

Lunch

Large tossed salad

4 teaspoons low-calorie salad dressing

2–4 oz (¼–½ cup) water-packed tuna

1 oz (½ medium) whole-wheat roll

Dinner

Large tossed salad

4 teaspoons low-calorie salad dressing

3 oz broiled lamb chop

2 oz (¼ small) baked sweet potato

1 teaspoon butter

Asparagus (as desired)

Add to or between meals 1 Milk Selection (see page 176) and 1 Fruit Selection (see pages 177–78).

DAY 9 GOURMET

Breakfast

* 3 Lean Line Corn Muffins

8 oz (1 cup) skim milk

Lunch

Large tossed salad

4 teaspoons low-calorie salad dressing

* Baked Stuffed Potato

Dinner

Large tossed salad

4 teaspoons low-calorie salad dressing

* Shrimp Boats

Add to or between meals 1 Fruit Selection (see pages 177–78).

DAY 9 GOURMET
RECIPES

▮ LEAN LINE CORN MUFFINS ▮
(3 muffins, or 1 serving) 320 calories

---

1 egg

⅓ cup nonfat dry milk (undissolved)

---

1 oz (2 tablespoons) corn meal

---

3 oz (⅓ cup) canned unsweetened, pineapple (crushed or in chunks), drained

---

1 oz (⅛ cup) juice reserved from canned pineapple

¼ teaspoon baking soda

Blend all ingredients in blender until mixed but not smooth. Spoon into 3 cupcake tins coated with no-stick vegetable cooking spray. Bake at 350° for 15–20 minutes, or until brown.

COUNTS AS: 1 Breakfast Protein List C *or* 1 Bonus List A Selection
1 Bread Selection
1 Fruit Selection
1 Milk Selection

∎ BAKED STUFFED POTATO ∎
270 calories

4 oz (1 very small) potato
1 oz (2 tablespoons) skim milk
1 oz (2 tablespoons) low-fat cottage cheese
2 oz (¼ cup) cooked broccoli
1½ oz (1½ slices) natural cheddar cheese
Salt, pepper, paprika, chives, and parsley to taste

Bake potato at 350°. When done, cut in half lengthwise and scoop out potato. Mash, and beat in skim milk. Mix in cottage cheese, broccoli, and cheddar cheese, and season. Refill potato shells with mixture and sprinkle with seasonings. Return to 350° oven and bake until top is browned (1–2 minutes).

COUNTS AS: 1 Lunch Protein List C
1 Vegetable List B Selection
⅛ Milk Selection

∎ SHRIMP BOATS ∎
330 calories

6 oz (¾ cup) canned, frozen, or fresh shrimp or water-packed tuna
1 large stalk celery, finely chopped
1 oz (2 tablespoons) finely chopped scallions
3 oz (⅓ cup) cooked elbow macaroni
2 teaspoons imitation mayonnaise
1 teaspoon freshly squeezed lemon juice
8 oz (1 medium) cucumber
Paprika to taste

In bowl, combine shrimp, celery, scallions, macaroni, mayonnaise, and lemon juice. Peel cucumber and score sides lengthwise with a fork. Cut in half lengthwise and scoop out seeds. Divide shrimp mixture equally into 2 portions. Fill each cucumber half with half of shrimp mixture. Sprinkle with paprika. Chill.

COUNTS AS: 1 Dinner Protein List B
¼ Vegetable List A Selection *or* ¼ Bonus List A Selection (onions)
1 Bread Selection
1 Oil and Condiment Selection

DAY 10 PLAIN

Breakfast

8 oz (½ medium) grapefruit
2 oz (¼ cup) low-fat cottage cheese
¾ oz (½ cup) bran flakes
2 tablespoons unprocessed bran
8 oz (1 cup) skim milk

Lunch

Large tossed salad
4 teaspoons low-calorie salad dressing
2–4 oz broiled veal burger
1 oz (½ medium) hard roll

Dinner

Large tossed salad
4 teaspoons low-calorie salad dressing
4–6 oz cooked white turkey meat

2 teaspoons gravy

4 oz (½ cup) cooked sliced carrots

Add to or between meals 1 Milk Selection (see page 176) and 1 Fruit Selection (see pages 177–78).

DAY 10 GOURMET

Breakfast

*Banana-Nut Bread

2 tablespoons unprocessed bran

6 oz (¾ cup) skim milk

Lunch

8 oz (½ medium) grapefruit

Large tossed salad

*Gourmet Hot Dogs

Dinner

Large tossed salad

4 teaspoons low-calorie salad dressing

*Beef Barbecue

3 oz (⅓ cup) cooked sliced carrots

Add to or between meals ½ Bread Selection (see page 175) and 1 Milk Selection (see page 176).

DAY 10 GOURMET
RECIPES

■ BANANA-NUT BREAD ■
(8 servings) 260 calories per serving

4 oz (1 cup) whole-wheat flour
2 oz (½ cup) wheat germ
⅔ cup nonfat dry milk
½ teaspoon salt
2½ teaspoons baking powder
2 oz (¼ cup) chopped mixed nuts
2 oz (¼ cup) chopped dates
2 tablespoons unprocessed bran
8 teaspoons corn or safflower oil
1 lb (2 cups) peeled and mashed bananas
2 eggs
½ teaspoon grated lemon rind

Combine first 8 ingredients. Add remaining ingredients, and stir for not more than 40 strokes. Coat loaf pan with no-stick vegetable cooking spray. Turn out banana mixture into pan and bake at 350° for about 1 hour. Cool.

EACH SERVING COUNTS AS: 1 Breakfast Protein combined Lists C and D
1 Bread Selection
1 Fruit Selection
¼ Milk Selection
1 Oil and Condiment Selection

▮ GOURMET HOT DOGS ▮
280 calories

1½ oz (1 medium) hot dot
5 small stuffed green olives, halved
½ oz (½ slice) bread
½ oz (½ slice) natural American cheese

Broil hot dog, slit lengthwise halfway through, and stuff with olives. Place on bread from corner to corner. Cover with cheese placed squarely over bread. Broil unil cheese melts. Fold side corners up around hot dog, and serve.

COUNTS AS: 1 Lunch Protein combined Lists A and C
½ Bread Selection
1 Oil and Condiment Selection

▮ BEEF BARBECUE ▮
350 calories

1 oz (2 tablespoons) coarsely chopped onions
1 large stalk celery, sliced
3 oz (1 medium) green pepper, sliced (optional)
4 oz (½ cup) water
3 oz (⅓ cup) cut-up leftover beef or other meat
4 oz (½ cup) tomato juice
2 tablespoons ketchup
1 teaspoon vinegar, salt, pepper, and basil

Place onions, celery, and green pepper in saucepan and add enough water to cover. Simmer ten minutes. Add remaining ingredients. Simmer until vegetables are tender.

COUNTS AS: 1 Dinner Protein List A
            ¼ Vegetable List A Selection
            1 Oil and Condiment Selection
            ½ Daily tomato juice from Free Food List

DAY 11 PLAIN

Breakfast

8 oz (½ medium) grapefruit

*1 egg scrambled with 1 teaspoon butter and
2 tablespoons unprocessed bran*

1 oz (1 slice) whole-wheat bread

Lunch

Large tossed salad

4 teaspoons low-calorie salad dressing

2 oz lean roast beef

1 oz (1 slice) rye bread

8 oz (1 cup) skim milk

Dinner

Large tossed salad

4 teaspoons low-calorie salad dressing

6 oz roast chicken

4 oz (½ medium) baked potato

*Add to or between meals 1 Milk Selection (see
page 176) and 1 Fruit Selection (see pages
177–78).*

DAY 11 GOURMET

Breakfast

8 oz (½ medium) grapefruit

1 oz (¼ cup) wheat germ

4 oz (½ cup) cooked oatmeal

2 tablespoons unprocessed bran

8 oz (1 cup) skim milk

Lunch

Large tossed salad

4 teaspoons low-calorie salad dressing

*Italian Cheese Soufflé

Dinner

Large tossed salad

4 teaspoons low-calorie salad dressing

*Ricotta-Stuffed Peppers

Green beans (as desired) with

1 teaspoon butter

Add to or between meals 1 Bread Selection (see page 175), 1 Milk Selection (see page 176), 1 Fruit Selection (see pages 177–78).

DAY 11 GOURMET
RECIPES

∎ ITALIAN CHEESE SOUFFLÉ ∎
195 calories

1 10-oz package frozen broccoli or 1¼ cups chopped fresh broccoli
2 oz (¼ cup) part-skim ricotta cheese
2 oz (¼ cup) canned sliced mushrooms, drained
⅛ teaspoon garlic powder
Sprinkling of fennel seeds
2 egg whites

Cook and drain broccoli. Mix with ricotta, mushrooms, and seasonings. Beat egg whites until stiff peaks form. Fold into broccoli mixture. Turn out into dish coated with no-stick vegetable cooking spray, and bake at 350° for 20 minutes, or until firm.

COUNTS AS: 1 Lunch Protein List C

∎ RICOTTA-STUFFED PEPPERS ∎
385 calories

3 oz (1 medium) green pepper
4 oz (½ cup) part-skim ricotta cheese
4 oz (½ cup) canned or fresh sliced mushrooms, drained,
Salt, pepper, and parsley to taste
4 oz (½ cup) home-style meatless oil-free tomato sauce
1 oz (2 tablespoons) grated Parmesan cheese

Wash green pepper, remove seeds, and parboil to soften. Mix together ricotta, mushrooms, and seasonings. Stuff pepper with ricotta mixture. Place in small baking pan. Pour tomato sauce over top and sprinkle with Parmesan cheese. Bake at 350° for 20–25 minutes, until heated through.

COUNTS AS: 1 Dinner Protein List C
1 Vegetable List A Selection

DAY 12 PLAIN

Breakfast

8 oz (1 cup) fresh strawberries
½ oz (1 tablespoon) chopped nuts
¾ oz (¾ cup) crispy rice cereal
2 tablespoons unprocessed bran
8 oz (1 cup) skim milk

Lunch

Large tossed salad
4 teaspoons low-calorie salad dressing
4 oz (½ cup) low-fat cottage cheese

Dinner

Large tossed salad
4 teaspoons low-calorie salad dressing
4–6 oz broiled flounder filet
3 oz (⅓ cup) cooked brown rice with
1 teaspoon butter

Add to or between meals 1 Milk Selection (see page 176) and 1 Fruit Selection (see pages 177–78).

DAY 12 GOURMET

Breakfast

*Banana Shake

Lunch

4 oz (½ cup) unsweetened grapefruit sections

Large tossed salad

4 teaspoons low-calorie salad dressing

*Toni's Yummy Sandwich Spread

1 oz (1 slice) rye bread

Dinner

Large tossed salad

4 teaspoons low-calorie salad dressing

*French Veal Patty au Poivre

*Pickled Beets

Add to or between meals 1 Bread Selection (see page 175), 1 Milk Selection (see page 176), and ½ Fruit Selection (see page 177–78).

DAY 12 GOURMET
RECIPES

▮ BANANA SHAKE ▮
210 calories

2 oz (¼ medium) banana, weighed with peel
8 oz (1 cup) skim milk
½ oz (1 tablespoon) peanut butter
2 ice cubes
2 tablespoons unprocessed bran

Peel banana. Mix together all ingredients in blender on high speed. Pour into tall glass. Drink immediately.

COUNTS AS: 1 Breakfast Protein List D *or* 1 Bonus List A Selection
½ Fruit Selection
1 Milk Selection

▮ TONI'S YUMMY SANDWICH SPREAD ▮
*90 calories (160 calories
with 1 Bread Selection)*

1 oz (⅛ cup) water-packed sardines, drained
2 oz (2 cup) low-fat cottage cheese
Salt to taste
1 teaspoon caraway seeds

Mix together all ingredients. Delicious spread on 1 Bread Selection.

COUNTS AS: 1 Lunch Protein combined Lists A and C
1 Bread Selection

❚ FRENCH VEAL PATTY AU POIVRE ❚
480 calories

7 oz (⅞ cup) lean ground veal (will cook down to 6 oz)
1 teaspoon coarsely ground black pepper
¼ teaspoon salt (optional)
1 teaspoon butter
1 teaspoon Tabasco sauce
1 teaspoon Worcestershire sauce
Freshly squeezed lemon juice to taste
Chopped fresh parsley and chives to taste

Shape veal lightly into patty, sprinkle each side with pepper (pressing pepper into meat), and let stand 30 minutes. Sprinkle light layer of salt into nonstick pan and place on high heat. When salt begins to brown, add veal patty. Cook until well browned on one side (about 10 minutes), turn, and cook until done, continually pouring off any accumulated fat. Transfer to plate. Add butter, Tabasco, Worcestershire, and lemon juice. Sprinkle with parsley and chives.

COUNTS AS: 1 Dinner Protein List B
　　　　　　1 Oil and Condiment Selection
　　　　　　⅔ Tabasco sauce from Free Food List

❚ PICKLED BEETS ❚
(2 servings) 50 calories per serving

8 oz (1 cup) cooked sliced, cubed or julienne beets, with juice
Onion flakes to taste
Artificial sweetener (to equal sweetness of 2 teaspoons sugar)
2 oz (¼ cup) cider vinegar

Mix together all ingredients and refrigerate. Ready to eat when chilled (may also be eaten warm if desired).

COUNTS AS: 1 Vegetable List A Selection

DAY 13 PLAIN

Breakfast

8 oz (½ medium) grapefruit
2 oz (¼ cup) part-skim ricotta cheese
¾ oz (½ cup) bran flakes
2 tablespoons unprocessed bran
8 oz (1 cup) skim milk

Lunch

Large tossed salad
4 teaspoons low-calorie salad dressing
2–4 oz (¼–½ cup) water-packed tuna
8 oz (1 cup) tomato juice

Dinner

Large tossed salad
4 teaspoons low-calorie salad dressing
4–6 oz cooked white turkey meat
2 teaspoons gravy
3 oz (⅓ cup) cooked brown rice
4 oz (½ cup) cooked green beans

Add to or between meals 1 Milk Selection (see page 176) and 1 Fruit Selection (see pages 177–78).

DAY 13 GOURMET

Breakfast

*Breakfast Jumble

8 oz (1 cup) skim milk

Lunch

Large tossed salad

4 teaspoons low-calorie salad dressing

*Broccoli-Rice Quiche

Dinner

Large tossed salad

4 teaspoons low-calorie salad dressing

3 oz lean roast beef

4 oz (½ cup) mashed butternut squash with

4 teaspoons sour cream

Add to or between meals 1 Milk Selection (see page 176) and 1 Fruit Selection (see pages 177–78).

DAY 13 GOURMET
RECIPES

▌ BREAKFAST JUMBLE ▌
170 calories

¾ oz (¾ cup) crispy rice cereal
2 oz (¼ cup) low-fat cottage cheese
4 oz (½ cup) fresh blueberries
Artificial sweetener (to equal sweetness of 2 teaspoons sugar)
Dash ground cinnamon
2 tablespoons unprocessed bran

Jumble together all ingredients in bowl. Enjoy! An easy, quick, and delicious breakfast.

COUNTS AS: 1 Breakfast Protein List C
1 Bread Selection
1 Fruit Selection

▌ BROCCOLI-RICE QUICHE ▌
(3 servings) 340 calories per serving

9 oz (1 cup) cooked enriched white rice
3 oz (6 tablespoons) grated Parmesan cheese
3 eggs
Salt to taste
3 oz (6 tablespoons) skim milk
6 oz (¾ cup) canned or fresh sliced mushrooms, drained
1 10-oz package frozen broccoli or 1¼ cups chopped fresh broccoli
Pepper to taste

Combine rice, half the grated cheese, 1 egg (slightly beaten), and salt in bowl; mix well. Then press firmly onto bottom of pie pan. Beat remaining eggs slightly, stirring in milk, mushrooms, broccoli, salt, and pepper. Spoon broccoli mixture over rice mixture. Bake at 370° for 20 minutes. Sprinkle with remaining cheese and bake 10 minutes longer.

COUNTS AS: 1 Lunch Protein List C
1 Bread Selection
⅛ Milk Selection *or* ⅛ Bonus List A Selection (milk)

DAY 14 PLAIN

Breakfast

8 oz (½ medium) grapefruit

1 egg scrambled with

2 tablespoons unprocessed bran

1 oz (1 slice) whole-wheat toast

1 teaspoon butter

Lunch

Large tossed salad

4 teaspoons low-calorie salad dressing

4 oz (½ cup) low-fat plain yogurt with

1 oz (2 tablespoons) chopped mixed nuts

Dinner

Large tossed salad

4 teaspoons low-calorie salad dressing

4–6 oz broiled Monk fish

3 oz (⅓ cup) cooked brown rice

4 oz (½ cup) cooked sliced asparagus

Add to or between meals 1 Milk Selection (see page 176) and 1 Fruit Selection (see pages 177–78).

DAY 14 GOURMET

Breakfast

8 oz (½ medium) grapefruit

* 2 Delicious Bran Muffins

1 teaspoon butter

8 oz (1 cup) skim milk

Lunch

Large tossed salad

4 teaspoons low-calorie salad dressing

1 hard-boiled egg

2 oz (¼ cup) water-packed tuna

8 oz (1 medium) orange

Dinner

Large tossed salad

4 teaspoons low-calorie salad dressing

*Beef Cubes in Gravy

1½ oz (3 tablespoons) cooked enriched white rice

Add to or between meals 1 Milk Selection (see page 176).

DAY 14 GOURMET
RECIPES

▮ DELICIOUS BRAN MUFFINS ▮
(6 muffins, or 3 servings)
150 calories per serving

2¼ oz (1⅛ cups) 100% bran cereal
3 eggs
Artificial sweetener (to equal sweetness of 6 teaspoons sugar)
¼ teaspoon salt
2 oz (¼ cup) water
1 teaspoon baking powder

Mix together all ingredients. Spoon equally into 6 nonstick muffin tins or muffin tins coated with no-stick vegetable cooking spray. Bake at 350° for 15–20 minutes.

2 MUFFINS COUNT AS: 1 Breakfast Protein List C
1 Bread Selection

▮ BEEF CUBES IN GRAVY ▮
280 calories

1 packet onion bouillon powder or 1 cube
1 packet beef bouillon
8 oz (1 cup) boiling water
1 tablespoon flour
3 oz (⅓ cup) cooked beef cubes
2 oz (¼ cup) canned or fresh sliced mushrooms
2 oz (½ medium) green pepper, diced

Dissolve onion and beef bouillon in 1 cup boiling water. Combine approximately a third of bouillon with flour. Shake until smooth. Pour remaining bouillon into saucepan. Add flour mixture and stir until smooth. Add beef cubes, mushrooms, and peppers. Heat through.

COUNTS AS: 1 Dinner Protein List A
½ Bread Selection

7.
PROGRAMMING
A PARTY—
WEEK 3

The Lean Line Program doesn't preclude a party—yours or someone else's. We want you to have fun. In the past, you probably went off your diet as soon as you stood before the bountiful buffet or sat at the bar.

Why? Was it the food that tempted you or was it because you wanted to be liked and felt that in order to be accepted you must eat? Were you convinced that you would offend someone if you refused food? The truth is that no one *really* notices what you eat or drink—they are too busy taking care of their own needs.

What about the host or hostess who constantly offers food and drink? The easiest way to solve that problem is with a "No, thank you. I don't eat that." Your reasons are your own. A host would not insist that a diabetic eat chocolate or that an alcoholic take a drink or that a person suffering from high blood pressure eat salty food. Let them assume you have a medical reason for not eating a particular food. You do! Obesity is a medical problem, and you have the right to refuse food.

Keep in mind that self-control does not mean standing in the face of temptation and then struggling to resist it. Self-control is a method of avoiding temptation by deciding ahead of time what the consequences of your actions will be so that you arrange your situation to avoid temptation.

As you dress for the party, think of yourself as thin. Dress like a thin person. If you have been losing weight, it is time to treat yourself to a new outfit. It will make you aware of your slimmer body and encourage you to stay on your One Month Lighter Program. Other people will also notice the new you, and there is nothing like a compliment to spur you on. Put your best foot forward even if the event is a backyard barbecue with comfortable old friends.

There is no need to test yourself unnecessarily. At a party, therefore, position yourself as far away from the food as possible. Most overweight people have a tendency to sit right next to the chips and dip or linger near the hors d'oeuvres. The closer you are to the snacks, the easier it will be to have "just one."

Holding a glass is a social custom. You probably will feel more comfortable with a glass in your hand at a party, and others attending will feel more comfortable with you. Liquor is a source of a lot of empty calories. It can sabotage many aspects of self-control. Why not take diet soda in a champagne glass, or a wine spritzer (seltzer and a little wine), or, of course, that famous drink of the jet set, mineral water with a twist of lime in it? If you still want hard liquor, take one drink and nurse it, or divide the shot between two glasses of water or seltzer. No one at the party will be keeping track of what's in your glass or how many you've had.

Once you've safely made your way through the cocktail hour, can you do the same for the meal? Of course you can, and you can do it unobtrusively and still enjoy yourself. Suppose the meal is served buffet-style. As we all have learned, a buffet offers unlimited temptations. The Roman gorgers never had it so good. But a big spread of choices offers just that—choices. Why not select the cut vegetables or the lean roast beef or turkey? Is the chicken salad squishy with mayonnaise better than just plain shrimp? Don't the fatty spare ribs look better than they taste? Why not some fruit instead of quiche, or, if you want cheese, a wedge of hard cheese would be a wiser selection than quiche.

Before you make your choices, ask yourself whether each food is worth it. If it is, won't a little do just as well as a heaping plateful? Aren't your eyes usually bigger than your stomach? Can't you always go back for seconds? If you can get away from the table, the chances are good that you can resist the effort to stand in line the second time, or you'll get distracted by good company and never make it back to the table.

Okay, suppose it is a sit-down dinner, where you are under the watchful eye of the hostess? How can you stick to your diet without insulting your hostess and making your dinner companions uneasy. First of all, you eat *very* slowly. Make a game out of being the last one finished. Put your fork down between bites and chew what is in your mouth completely. You won't have to refuse seconds if you are still on your firsts.

Don't eat everything on your plate. Remember, it is the first taste that's best anyway.

When the party's over and you've successfully resisted your old fat behaviors, don't let it go to your head—or waist. Don't go home and reward yourself for being so good with a "little snack." Go to bed and dream of the new you.

Soon, you won't even have to think twice about what to eat at a party. Your selection of the "right stuff" will have become automatic because that will be the way you always eat at home.

Now, here is your third week of the One Month Lighter Lean Line Program. As you can see, many of the recipes can be used when you want to entertain in your own home. Your friends—fat or thin—will enjoy the meals and be grateful for the controlled calories, good taste, and ample nutrition.

DAY 15 PLAIN

Breakfast

8 oz (1 cup) fresh strawberries

1 egg scrambled with 2 teaspoons imitation margarine and 2 tablepoons unprocessed bran

1 oz (¾ small) corn muffin

8 oz (1 cup) skim milk

Lunch

Large tossed salad

4 teaspoons low-calorie salad dressing

2–4 oz (¼–½ cup) cold cooked shrimp

1 oz (½ medium) hard roll

Dinner

Large tossed salad

4 teaspoons low-calorie salad dressing

3 oz broiled lamb chop

4 oz (½ cup) mashed butternut squash

Add to or between meals 1 Milk Selection (see page 176) and 1 Fruit Selection (see pages 177–78).

DAY 15 GOURMET

Breakfast

8 oz (1 medium) orange

1 egg scrambled with 2 tablespoons unprocessed bran

1 strip bacon

Lunch

* Salad in a Pocket

8 oz (1 cup) skim milk

Dinner

Large tossed salad

4 teaspoons low-calorie salad dressing

* Scallops Cacciatore

3 oz (⅓ cup) cooked spaghetti

Add to or between meals 1 Milk Selection (see page 176) and 1 Fruit Selection (see pages 177–78).

DAY 15 GOURMET
RECIPES

▮ SALAD IN A POCKET ▮
365 calories

1 oz (1 small or ½ large) pita bread
1 oz (1 slice) natural American or cheddar cheese, shredded
2 oz (2 slices) turkey, shredded
Lettuce, shredded (as desired)
2 oz (¼ medium) cucumber, diced
2 oz (½ medium) tomato, diced
1 teaspoon vegetable oil
1 teaspoon vinegar

Split bread and fill with remaining ingredients.

COUNTS AS: 1 Lunch Protein combined Lists B and C
1 Bread Selection
1 Oil and Condiment Selection

▌ SCALLOPS CACCIATORE ▌
415 calories

4 oz (½ cup) tomato juice
1 clove garlic, minced
1 teaspoon salt
4 peppercorns, crushed
1 tablespoon wine vinegar
Sprinkling of onion flakes
3 oz (1 medium) green pepper, cut into strips
4 oz (½ cup) sliced fresh mushrooms
8 oz (1 cup) scallops (will cook down to 6 oz)
2 oz (¼ cup) freshly squeezed lemon juice

Combine first 6 ingredients in saucepan. Cook covered over moderate heat for 5 minutes. Remove from heat. Add green pepper and mushrooms. Put scallops in baking dish and pour lemon juice over them. Bake uncovered at 350° for 10 minutes. Remove from oven and drain off lemon juice. Add saucepan mixture to scallops and bake a few minutes longer.

COUNTS AS: 1 Dinner Protein List B
½ Daily tomato juice from Free Food List

DAY 16 PLAIN

Breakfast

4 oz (½ medium) banana, weighed with peel
½ oz (1 tablespoon) chopped mixed nuts
4 oz (½ cup) cooked oatmeal
2 tablespoons unprocessed bran
8 oz (1 cup) skim milk

Lunch

Large tossed salad
4 teaspoons low-calorie salad dressing
2 hard-boiled eggs
1 oz (1 slice) whole-wheat bread
8 oz (1 cup) tomato juice

Dinner

Large tossed salad
4 teaspoons low-calorie salad dressing
4–6 oz broiled filet of sole
4 oz (½ medium) baked potato with
4 teaspoons sour cream

Add to or between meals 1 Milk Selection (see page 176) and 1 Fruit Selection (see pages 177–78).

DAY 16 GOURMET

Breakfast

8 oz (½ medium) grapefruit
1 soft-boiled egg
¾ oz (¾ cup) cornflakes
2 tablespoons unprocessed bran
8 oz (1 cup) skim milk

Lunch

* Fruit Salad Luncheon

Dinner

Large tossed salad

---

4 teaspoons low-calorie salad dressing

---

* Baked Chicken

---

4 oz (½ cup) cooked sliced carrots

---

4 oz (½ cup) cooked green beans

Add to or between meals: 4 oz (½ cup) low-fat plain yogurt and 1 oz (2 tablespoons) chopped mixed nuts.

DAY 16 GOURMET RECIPES

▌ FRUIT SALAD LUNCHEON ▌
180 calories

---

1 package sugar-free orange-flavored gelatin

---

4 oz (½ cup) low-fat cottage cheese or part-skim ricotta cheese

---

4 oz (½ cup) canned peaches, packed in own juice, drained

Prepare gelatin according to package directions. When practically set, add remaining ingredients. Refrigerate until firm.

COUNTS AS: 1 Lunch Protein List C
            1 Fruit Selection

▮ BAKED CHICKEN ▮
360 calories

1 oz (1 slice) bread, cubed
1 oz (2 tablespoons) diced onions
1 oz (2 tablespoons) diced celery
Salt and pepper to taste
1 packet chicken bouillon or 1 chicken bouillon cube dissolved in 8 oz (1 cup) water
4–6 oz (½–¾ cup) cubed cooked chicken

Combine bread, onions, celery, salt, and pepper. Moisten vegetables with 4 oz (½ cup) bouillon. (Discard remaining bouillon.) Place chicken in nonstick pan or pan sprayed with no-stick vegetable cooking spray. Cover with bread mixture. Bake, covered, at 350° for 1 hour.

COUNTS AS: 1 Dinner Protein List B
¼ Vegetable List A Selection
1 Bread Selection

DAY 17 PLAIN

Breakfast

8 oz (½ medium) grapefruit
2 oz (¼ cup) low-fat cottage cheese
¾ oz (1½ cups) puffed rice
2 tablespoons unprocessed bran
8 oz (1 cup) skim milk

Lunch

Large tossed salad

4 teaspoons low-calorie salad dressing

2–4 oz baked chicken

4 oz (½ cup) cooked sliced asparagus

1 teaspoon butter

Dinner

Large tossed salad

4 teaspoons low-calorie salad dressing

3 oz lean roast beef

3 oz (⅓ cup) cooked enriched white rice

4 oz (½ cup) whole-kernel corn

Add to or between meals 1 Milk Selection (see page 176) and 1 Fruit Selection (see pages 177–78).

DAY 17 GOURMET

Breakfast

*Julie's Crunchy Bar

Lunch

Large tossed salad

4 teaspoons low-calorie salad dressing

4 oz (½ cup) water-packed tuna

Dinner

Large tossed salad
4 teaspoons low-calorie salad dressing
* Shrimp Jambalaya
Add to or between meals 1 Milk Selection (see page 176) and 1 Fruit Selection (see pages 177–78).

DAY 17 GOURMET RECIPES

❚ JULIE'S CRUNCHY BAR ❚
365 calories

¾ oz (¾ cup) cornflakes
1 packet low-calorie hot cocoa mix, undissolved
½ oz (1 tablespoon) raisins
½ oz (1 tablespoon) chopped mixed nuts
1 teaspoon vanilla extract
1 egg
Artificial sweetener (to equal sweetness of 2 teaspoons sugar)

Mix together all ingredients. Transfer to small pan coated with no-stick vegetable cooking spray or to nonstick pan. Bake in 350° oven for ½ hour. Chill and serve.

COUNTS AS: 1 Breakfast Protein List D
1 Bread Selection
1 Fruit Selection
1 Milk Selection
1 Oil and Condiment Selection

▮ SHRIMP JAMBALAYA ▮
440 calories

8 oz (1 cup) tomato juice or vegetable juice cocktail
2 oz (4 tablespoons) chopped green pepper
2 oz (4 tablespoons) chopped celery
2 oz (¼ cup) minced onions
2 oz (¼ cup) canned tomatoes
Garlic powder, chili powder, salt, and pepper to taste
3 oz (3 slices) turkey ham, shredded
3 oz (⅓ cup) cooked shrimp
3 oz (⅓ cup) cooked enriched white rice

In large saucepan, combine all ingredients except meat, shrimp, and rice. Cook mixture covered over medium heat until vegetables are tender. Add turkey ham and shrimp. Heat and serve warm over cooked rice.

COUNTS AS: 1 Dinner Protein combined Lists A and B
½ Vegetable List A Selection
1 Bread Selection
Daily tomato juice from Free Food List

DAY 18 PLAIN

Breakfast

8 oz (½ medium) grapefruit
1 oz (¼ cup) wheat germ
4 oz (½ cup) cooked farina
2 tablespoons unprocessed bran
8 oz (1 cup) skim milk

Lunch

Large tossed salad

4 teaspoons low-calorie salad dressing

2 oz broiled hamburger

1 oz (½ medium) rye roll

2 tablespoons ketchup

Dinner

Large tossed salad

4 teaspoons low-calorie salad dressing

4–6 oz (½–¾ cup) broiled scallops

4 oz (½ small) cooked acorn squash

Add to or between meals 1 Milk Selection (see page 176) and 1 Fruit Selection (see pages 177–78).

DAY 18 GOURMET

Breakfast

* Cranberry-Walnut Muffin

8 oz (1 cup) skim milk

Lunch

Large tossed salad

2 oz lean roast beef

4 teaspoons low-calorie salad dressing

12 oz (½ small) cantaloupe

Dinner

* Tomato Soup

* Curried Turkey and Sprouts

Add to or between meals 1 Milk Selection (see page 176) and ¾ Fruit Selection (see pages 177–78).

DAY 18 GOURMET RECIPES

❚ CRANBERRY-WALNUT MUFFIN ❚
(8 servings) 175 calories per muffin

4 oz (1 cup) flour

4 oz (1 cup) wheat germ

½ teaspoon baking soda

1½ teaspoons baking powder

Artificial sweetener (to equal sweetness of 4 teaspoons sugar)

1 teaspoon grated orange rind

1½ oz (3 tablespoons) chopped walnuts

1 egg

4 oz (½ cup) orange juice

4 teaspoons vegetable oil

4 oz (1 cup) halved fresh cranberries

Combine first 7 ingredients. Separately, combine egg, juice, and oil. Add to dry ingredients and mix well. Fold in cranberries. Spoon mixture into 8 nonstick muffin tins or muffin tins coated with no-stick vegetable cooking spray and bake at 350° for 20 minutes.

1 MUFFIN COUNTS AS: 1 Breakfast Protein List D
1 Bread Selection
¼ Fruit Selection
1 Oil and Condiment Selection

❙ TOMATO SOUP ❙
106 calories

8 oz (1 cup) tomato juice
4 oz (½ cup) sliced fresh mushrooms
Salt and pepper to taste
2 teaspoons imitation margarine

Mix together all ingredients in saucepan. Heat thoroughly over medium heat and serve.

COUNTS AS: 1 Oil and Condiment Selection
Daily tomato juice from Free Food List

❙ CURRIED TURKEY AND SPROUTS ❙
465 calories

1 packet chicken bouillon powder or 1 bouillon cube
8 oz (1 cup) boiling water
2 tablespoons flour
2 oz (½ cup) bean sprouts
2 oz (¼ cup) sliced carrots
2 oz (¼ cup) sliced onions
4 oz (½ cup) chopped green pepper
4 oz (½ cup) sliced celery
6 oz (¾ cup) diced cooked white turkey meat
¼ teaspoon curry powder

In large saucepan, empty chicken bouillon into 1 cup boiling water. Stir in flour and cook until thickened. Add vegetables and simmer for 10 minutes, or until vegetables are tender. Add turkey and curry powder, and heat thoroughly.

EACH SERVING COUNTS AS: 1 Dinner Protein List B
                                      1 Vegetable List A Selection
                                      1 Bread Selection

DAY 19 PLAIN

Breakfast

4 oz (½ cup) grapefruit juice

1 soft-boiled egg

¾ oz (¾ cup) crispy rice cereal

2 tablespoons unprocessed bran

8 oz (1 cup) skim milk

Lunch

Large tossed salad

4 teaspoons low-calorie salad dressing

2–4 oz broiled filet of sole

1 teaspoon butter

4 oz (½ cup) cooked sliced carrots

8 oz (1 cup) fresh strawberries

Dinner

Large tossed salad

4 teaspoons low-calorie salad dressing

3 oz broiled lamb chop

3 oz (⅓ cup) cooked brown rice

4 oz (½ cup) cooked sliced zucchini

Add to or between meals 1 Milk Selection (see page 176).

DAY 19 GOURMET

Breakfast

* Baked Apple Slices

1 oz (1 slice) natural cheddar cheese

8 oz (1 cup) skim milk

Lunch

Large tossed salad

4 teaspoons low-calorie salad dressing

* Stuffed Pepper Texas-Style

Dinner

Large tossed salad

4 teaspoons low-calorie salad dressing

* Chow Mein

1 oz (½ medium) roll (omit if rice or matzo is eaten with Chow Mein)

1 teaspoon butter

Add to or between meals 1 Milk Selection (see page 176) and 1 Fruit Selection (see pages 177–78).

DAY 19 GOURMET RECIPES

▌ BAKED APPLE SLICES ▌
80 calories

---

4 oz (1 medium) apple, unpeeled, cored, and thinly sliced

Sprinkling of ground cinnamon or nutmeg

Artificial sweetener (to equal sweetness of 2 teaspoons sugar)

Sprinkle apple slices with cinnamon and sweetener. Reassemble apple. Place on piece of aluminum foil and wrap tightly. Bake at 350° for about 20 minutes, or until tender.

COUNTS AS: 1 Fruit Selection

▌ STUFFED PEPPER TEXAS-STYLE ▌
385 calories

---

3 oz (1 medium) green pepper

---

4 oz (½ cup) sliced mushrooms

---

1 oz (½ cup) chopped fresh spinach

1½ teaspoons soy sauce

---

3 oz (⅓ cup) cooked enriched white rice

---

2 oz (2 slices) natural cheddar cheese, diced

Seasonings to taste

Wash pepper, remove top and seeds, and parboil until tender. In wok or saucepan stir-fry mushrooms and spinach in soy sauce. Add cooked rice. Let cool. Mix in cheddar cheese and seasonings. Stuff pepper with rice mixture and bake at 350° for 20 minutes.

COUNTS AS: 1 Lunch Protein List C
1 Bread Selection
½ Daily soy sauce from Free Food List

∎ CHOW MEIN ∎
475 calories

2–4 oz (½–1 cup) bean sprouts
2 oz (¼ cup) diced water chestnuts
2 oz (¼ cup) sliced onions
4 oz (½ cup) sliced celery
2 oz (¼ cup) sliced fresh mushrooms (optional)
1½ teaspoons soy sauce
Salt and pepper to taste
6 oz (¾ cup) cubed cooked chicken

In large nonstick skillet or skillet coated with no-stick vegetable cooking spray, sauté vegetables, soy sauce, salt, and pepper until celery is tender-crisp. Add chicken and heat uncovered a few minutes longer. Serve. This may be served over 3 oz (⅓ cup) cooked rice or ¾ oz (½ cup) crumbled matzo, instead of eaten with dinner roll.

COUNTS AS: 1 Dinner Protein List B
1 Vegetable List A Selection
1 Bread Selection (if rice or matzo is used)
½ Daily soy sauce from Free Food List

DAY 20 PLAIN

Breakfast

8 oz (½ medium) grapefruit

1 oz (1 slice) natural hard cheese

¾ oz (1½ cups) puffed rice

2 tablespoons unprocessed bran

8 oz (1 cup) skim milk

Lunch

Spinach salad (as desired)

4 teaspoons low-calorie salad dressing

2–4 oz cooked white turkey meat

1 oz (½ medium) roll

1 teaspoon imitation margarine

8 oz (1 cup) skim milk

Dinner

Large tossed salad

4 teaspoons low-calorie salad dressing

3 oz broiled liver

4 oz (½ medium) baked potato with

2 teaspoons sour cream

Add to or between meals 1 Fruit Selection (see pages 177–78).

DAY 20 GOURMET

Breakfast

8 oz (1 cup) fresh strawberries

1 oz (1 slice) natural hard cheese

1 oz (½ medium) English muffin

Lunch

Large tossed salad

4 teaspoons low-calorie salad dressing

* Coconut-Pineapple Creamy Cheesecake

Dinner

Large tossed salad

4 teaspoons low-calorie salad dressing

* Shrimp Scampi

3 oz (⅓ cup) cooked enriched white rice

Add to or between meals ½ Milk Selection (see page 176) and 1 Oil and Condiment Selection (see page 179).

DAY 20 GOURMET
RECIPES

▮ COCONUT-PINEAPPLE CREAMY
CHEESECAKE ▮
235 calories

1 envelope unflavored gelatin
2 tablespoons cold water
4 oz (½ cup) boiling water
⅓ cup nonfat dry milk, undissolved
½ teaspoon pineapple extract
½ teaspoon coconut extract
Artificial sweetener to taste
4 oz (½ cup) low-fat cottage cheese
5 large ice cubes
4 oz (½ cup) well-drained canned unsweetened crushed pineapple

Place gelatin in blender. Add cold water and blend on low. Then add boiling water, dry milk, pineapple extract, coconut extract, and artificial sweetener. Blend on low. Next add cottage cheese and blend well. Then add ice cubes one at a time, blending after each addition. Stir in crushed pineapple and blend until mixed. Pour into mold. Put in freezer for 5 minutes, or until set. Store in refrigerator to eat later, or unmold immediately and eat the *whole* thing!

COUNTS AS: 1 Lunch Protein List C
1 Fruit Selection
1 Milk Selection

▮ SHRIMP SCAMPI ▮
200 calories

8 oz (1 cup) raw jumbo shrimp (will cook down to 6 oz)
4 oz (½ cup) buttermilk
¼ teaspoon salt
3 cloves garlic, crushed
2 teaspoons parsley flakes
1 teaspoon grated lemon peel
1 tablespoon freshly squeezed lemon juice
Lemon wedges (optional)

Shell and devein shrimp, except for tails. Wash shrimp under running water; then drain, pat dry with paper towels, and set aside. In bowl, mix together buttermilk, salt, garlic, parsley, lemon peel, and lemon juice. Arrange shrimp in shallow baking dish and cover with buttermilk mixture. Let stand for 10 minutes before baking. Bake at 400° for about 15 minutes, until fork-tender, or until shrimp are rosy pink. Arrange on platter and garnish with lemon wedges.

COUNTS AS: 1 Dinner Protein List B
½ Milk Selection

DAY 21 PLAIN

Breakfast

8 oz (½ medium) grapefruit
1 soft-boiled egg
¾ oz (⅓ cup) 100% bran cereal
2 tablespoons unprocessed bran
8 oz (1 cup) skim milk

Lunch

Large tossed salad

4 teaspoons low-calorie salad dressing

2–4 oz cooked white turkey meat

1 oz (1 slice) whole-wheat bread

1 teaspoon mayonnaise

Dinner

8 oz (1 cup) tomato juice

4–6 oz broiled filet of sole

4 oz (½ cup) sliced green beans

4 oz (½ cup) sliced tomatoes

1 teaspoon butter

Add to or between meals 1 Milk Selection (see page 176) and 1 Fruit Selection (see pages 177–78).

DAY 21 GOURMET

Breakfast

4 oz (½ medium) banana, weighed with peel

½ oz (1 tablespoon) chopped mixed nuts

¾ oz (½ cup) bran flakes

5 oz (⅝ cup) skim milk

Lunch

Large tossed salad

4 teaspoons low-calorie salad dressing

* Baked Beef Luncheon with Rice

Dinner

---

* *Chick-Pea Patties*

---

4 oz (½ medium) baked white potato with 1 teaspoon sour cream

---

Broccoli (as desired)

---

4 oz (½ cup) unsweetened orange sections

Add to or between meals 1 Milk Selection (see page 176).

DAY 21 GOURMET
RECIPES

▌ BAKED BEEF LUNCHEON WITH RICE ▐
(2 servings) 250 calories per serving

---

4 oz (½ cup) leftover chopped lean roast beef

---

6 oz (⅔ cup) cooked enriched white rice

---

1 beaten egg

---

4 oz (½ cup) skim milk

---

1 tablespoon imitation margarine

---

1 teaspoon chopped onions

½ teaspoon salt

Pepper to taste

Combine all ingredients. Place in small casserole coated with no-stick vegetable cooking spray. Bake uncovered at 350° for 40 minutes.

EACH SERVING COUNTS AS: 1 Lunch Protein combined Lists A and C
1 Bread Selection
¼ Milk Selection
¾ Oil and Condiment Selection

▮ CHICK-PEA PATTIES ▮
350 calories

6 oz (¾ cup) chick-peas (also called garbanzos)
1 oz (2 tablespoons) skim milk
1 tablespoon chopped fresh parsley
½ teaspoon ground cumin
½ teaspoon Worcestershire sauce
¼ teaspoon chili powder
¼ teaspoon dry mustard
4 teaspoons sour cream or 2 teaspoons imitation margarine

In large bowl, mash chick-peas with fork. Add remaining ingredients and mix well. (You may want to use hand mixer on low speed for more thorough blending.) Shape mixture into 3 patties and brown on each side in nonstick frying pan or frying pan coated with no-stick vegetable cooking spray. Five minutes on each side should be sufficient cooking time. Top patties with sour cream or imitation margarine and serve.

COUNTS AS: 1 Dinner Protein List D
⅛ Milk Selection
1 Oil and Condiment Selection

8. TRAVELING LIGHT— WEEK 4

Lillian Lawrence was so exact about sticking to her Lean Line Program when she traveled to Europe, she almost landed in a French prison. She took her nonfat dry milk with her, as the Lean Line Program suggests (see page 133), but she divided it up into little plastic sandwich bags. Guess what it looked like to French customs officials?

Eating out at a restaurant or traveling to the ends of the earth, you can maintain your food program.

The business lunch, for example, is a tradition in America, and it can be a diet destroyer, especially if you are under tension and dining with strangers. If you feel tense before a business lunch or dinner, we suggest that you go into the rest room and practice a relaxation technique, even if it's just stretching. Before the meal arrives drink a glass of water to make yourself feel fuller.

132 ONE MONTH LIGHTER

Of course, practice the Lean Line habit of chewing slowly and putting down your fork between bites. This makes the meal more satisfying and is conducive to good conversation.

Order a large salad. The real trick is to keep your mouth moving during a tense business lunch. If you get oral satisfaction from salad, you're safer.

If you must drink to be sociable—and this is less and less mandatory—order a jigger of whiskey, which is 107 calories, or a 12-oz glass of light beer (about 90 calories). You can nurse a glass of beer longer. A Virgin Mary (spicy tomato juice without the liquor) is better still. If you want a Bloody Mary (spicy tomato juice with the liquor), order two glasses of the mix and one shot of vodka to split between them. A glass of white wine (80 calories for 3 oz) or a spritzer of white wine and club soda are also good low-calorie choices.

For the main course you can select roasted, baked, grilled, or broiled lean meats or poultry. Avoid casseroles and dishes with gravies and sauces. Ask for oil and vinegar for your tossed salad and add them sparingly. For dessert, you can order fresh fruit.

A number of our members carry their tiny postal scales into the restaurant to weigh their food. We were accused once by the restaurant owner of being from the State Weights and Measures Division.

Overweight people are frequently nonassertive. Remember, we all have the right to order food prepared the way we wish in a restaurant. If the food is not prepared the way you specified, send it back. Do not succumb to the waiter's pressure.

A service person's tip depends on pleasing you, so they will usually be accommodating. Be specific when placing your order. Decide in advance what you will order and don't even look at the menu. You may be tempted to order the wrong thing if you do.

Food on the road and in hotels also may sabotage your food plan, unless you are clever. If you must eat fast food, choose reasonable items, such as selections from the salad bar, but watch the foods with mayonnaise, particularly the pasta and chicken salads, as they may be high in calories. Avoid hot dogs, hamburgers, and french fries. These are high in salt, fat, and cholesterol.

We suggest taking with you on the road a Lean Line Survival Kit, which Lillian Lawrence (the notorious milk trafficker) uses during her many travels. Besides the nonfat dry milk, we suggest:

- A can of evaporated skim milk to use as a substitute for local milk and cream.
- Diet sweetener.
- Fresh fruit or canned fruit (without sugar).
- Canned tuna and a can opener.
- Bouillon cubes and a heating coil that you place in the cup to heat up the liquid.
- Canned vegetables.
- Seltzer, mineral water, or diet soda.
- Cucumbers, carrots, celery, lettuce, and the like.

If you are traveling on a plane, telephone ahead to the airline and request your special meal. Edith Van Cleve was a little nervous about flying in a small plane. She was glad her suitcase containing her Lean Line Survival Kit fell within the allowable weight limit, but she gulped when the pilot asked her how much *she* weighed. She lied by about thirty pounds and then went to her seat. The small plane took off and then, instead of leaving the airport, kept circling. After about six circles, Edith struggled up to the pilot's door, rapped, and said, "I lied. I really weigh thirty pounds more than I said." Edith thought the weight on the plane was the problem when it was really just a short in the electrical system. Which only goes to show that you carry more than weight around with you on a trip—guilt is in the package.

If traveling by train, leave your guilt at home and bring your own food, or if there is a dining car, you can usually order broiled meats, fish, or poultry.

Now that you are about to begin your fourth week of the One Month Lighter Program, you've traveled a good way and we hope you've enjoyed the trip. The recipes and methods of cooking and eating should have become by now a part of your permanent "equipment." So keep on trucking! (We've included two extra days in the menu plan to round out the month.)

DAY 22 PLAIN

Breakfast

8 oz (½ medium) grapefruit
1 oz (¼ cup) wheat germ
4 oz (½ cup) cooked farina
2 tablespoons unprocessed bran
8 oz (1 cup) skim milk

Lunch

Large tossed salad
4 teaspoons low-calorie salad dressing
4 oz (½ cup) low-fat cottage cheese
4 oz (½ cup) cooked sliced green beans
4 oz (½ cup) sliced peaches, unsweetened canned or fresh

Dinner

Large spinach salad

4 teaspoons low-calorie salad dressing

3 oz broiled lamb chop

2 oz (¼ cup) baked beans

1 oz (½ medium) roll

1 teaspoon butter

Add to or between meals 1 Milk Selection (see page 176) and 1 Bread Selection (see page 175).

DAY 22 GOURMET

Breakfast

8 oz (½ medium) grapefruit

* 3 Zucchini Muffins

Lunch

Large tossed salad

4 teaspoons low-calorie salad dressing

2–4 oz (¼–½ cup) water-packed tuna

1 oz (½ large) whole-wheat pita bread

2 teaspoons imitation mayonnaise

Chopped celery to taste

Dinner

Large tossed salad

4 teaspoons low-calorie salad dressing

* Eggplant and Veal, prepared with Lean Line Tomato Sauce

Add to or between meals 1 Milk Selection (see page 176) and 1 Fruit Selection (see pages 177–78).

DAY 22 GOURMET RECIPES

▮ ZUCCHINI MUFFINS ▮
(12 muffins, or 4 servings)
150 calories per serving

2½ oz (1⅓ cups) 100% bran cereal

3 teaspoons baking powder

Artificial sweetener (to equal sweetness of 8 teaspoons sugar)

4 eggs

8 oz (1 cup) skim milk

2 teaspoons vanilla extract

2 cups drained cooked fresh zucchini

Combine cereal, baking powder, and sweetener. Blend eggs, skim milk, vanilla, and zucchini in blender. Then by hand mix together all ingredients until smooth. Let stand 5 minutes. Spoon into nonstick muffin tins or muffin tins coated with no-stick vegetable cooking spray. Bake at 350° for 20–25 minutes.

3 MUFFINS COUNT AS: 1 Breakfast Protein List C *or* Bonus
List A Selection
1 Bread Selection
1 Milk Selection

▮ EGGPLANT AND VEAL ▮
405 calories

4 oz (½ cup) peeled and sliced eggplant
6 oz (¾ cup) cooked ground veal
2 oz (1 small) green pepper, diced
Salt, pepper, and onion powder to taste
4 oz (½ cup) Lean Line Tomato Sauce (see page 197)
Basil to taste

Place eggplant in baking dish. Top with veal. Add green pepper
on top of veal layer and sprinkle with salt, pepper, and onion
powder. Pour tomato sauce over all and sprinkle with basil. Bake
covered at 375° for approximately 30 minutes.

COUNTS AS: 1 Dinner Protein List B

DAY 23 PLAIN

Breakfast

8 oz (½ medium) grapefruit
1 egg scrambled without butter or margarine
¾ oz (¾ cup) crispy rice cereal
2 tablespoons unprocessed bran
8 oz (1 cup) skim milk

Lunch

Large tossed salad

4 teaspoons low-calorie salad dressing

2–4 oz (¼–½ cup) cooked crab meat

1 oz (1 slice) rye bread

1 teaspoon mayonnaise

Dinner

Large tossed salad

4 teaspoons low-calorie salad dressing

4–6 oz broiled swordfish

4 oz (½ cup) cooked sliced beets

4 oz (½ cup) cooked chopped broccoli

Add to or between meals 1 Milk Selection (see page 176) and 1 Fruit Selection (see pages 177–78).

DAY 23 GOURMET

Breakfast

8 oz (½ medium) grapefruit

* 2 Bran Muffins

8 oz (1 cup) skim milk

Lunch

Large tossed salad

4 teaspoons low-calorie salad dressing

* Spanish Omelet

1 oz (1 slice) toasted whole-grain bread

1 teaspoon butter

Dinner

Large tossed salad

4 teaspoons low-calorie salad dressing

* Lemon Herbed Rock Cornish Hens

8 oz (1 cup) fresh strawberries

Add to or between meals 1 Milk Selection (see page 176).

DAY 23 GOURMET RECIPES

▮ BRAN MUFFINS ▮
(6 muffins, or 3 servings) 110 calories per serving

2 oz (1 cup) 100% bran cereal

2 teaspoons baking powder

Artificial sweetener (to equal sweetness of 6 teaspoons sugar)

3 eggs

2 teaspoons vanilla extract

3 oz (⅓ cup) water

Combine cereal, baking powder, and sweetener, and mix well. Add eggs, vanilla, and water. Mix until smooth. Let stand 5 minutes. Spoon into 6 nonstick muffin tins or muffin tins coated with no-stick vegetable cooking spray. Bake at 350° for 15–20 minutes.

2 MUFFINS COUNT AS: 1 Breakfast Protein List C *or* 1 Bonus
                    List A Selection
                    1 Bread Selection

▌ SPANISH OMELET ▌
220 calories

6 oz (¾ cup) tomato juice
2 oz (¼ cup) fresh or frozen French-style string beans
2 oz (¼ cup) sliced fresh or canned mushrooms
1 oz (¼ medium) green pepper, sliced very thin
Onion flakes, salt, and pepper to taste
2 eggs
1 tablespoon water

In skillet, cook uncovered tomato juice, vegetables, and seasonings until vegetables are tender. Make omelet of 2 eggs and water in nonstick skillet or skillet coated with no-stick vegetable cooking spray. Place vegetable filling on top and fold over as a regular omelet.

COUNTS AS: 1 Lunch Protein List C
¾ Daily tomato juice from Free Food List

▌ LEMON HERBED ROCK CORNISH HENS ▌
(4 servings) 335 calories per serving

2 20-oz Rock Cornish hens, split and skinned (will cook down to 6 oz per serving)
1 teaspoon garlic salt
¾ teaspoon coarsely ground black pepper
½ teaspoon paprika
½ teaspoon onion powder
3 tablespoons chopped fresh parsley
½ teaspoon dried rosemary
2 oz (¼ cup) freshly squeezed lemon juice

Sprinkle hens with seasonings. Place on rack in pan and pour lemon juice over hens. Bake at 325° for 1 hour, turning once during baking.

EACH SERVING COUNTS AS: 1 Dinner Protein List B

DAY 24 PLAIN

Breakfast

8 oz (½ medium) grapefruit

½ oz (1 tablespoon) chopped mixed nuts

4 oz (½ cup) cooked farina

2 tablespoons unprocessed bran

8 oz (1 cup) skim milk

Lunch

Large spinach salad

4 teaspoons low-calorie salad dressing

2–4 oz broiled veal burger

1 oz (½ medium) hard roll

2 tablespoons ketchup

8 oz (1 cup) skim milk

Dinner

8 oz (1 cup) tomato juice

Large tossed salad

4 teaspoons low-calorie salad dressing

3 oz broiled pork chop

2 oz (¼ small) baked sweet potato

Add to or between meals 1 Fruit Selection (see pages 177–78).

DAY 24 GOURMET

Breakfast

8 oz (1 cup) fresh strawberries

2 oz (¼ cup) part-skim ricotta cheese

1 oz (¾ small) corn muffin

2 teaspoons imitation margarine

8 oz (1 cup) low-calorie hot chocolate, made with artificial sweetener and skim milk

Lunch

Large tossed salad

4 teaspoons low-calorie salad dressing

* Broccoli Florentine

3 oz (⅓ cup) cooked enriched white rice

Dinner

Large tossed salad

4 teaspoons low-calorie salad dressing

* Salmon Croquettes

4 oz (½ cup) cooked sliced zucchini

4 oz (½ cup) cooked cauliflowerets

Add to or between meals 1 Milk Selection (see page 176) and 1 Fruit Selection (see pages 177–78).

DAY 24 GOURMET
RECIPES

▌ BROCCOLI FLORENTINE ▌
330 calories

---

1 10-oz package frozen broccoli or 1¼ cups chopped fresh broccoli

---

4 oz (½ cup) part-skim ricotta cheese

Salt, pepper, and parsley to taste

---

4 oz (½ cup) canned or fresh sliced mushrooms, drained

---

4 oz (½ cup) home-style meatless oilfree tomato sauce

Steam broccoli and drain. Mix ricotta with salt, pepper, and parsley. Then mix together broccoli, mushrooms, and seasoned ricotta. Turn out into small casserole coated with no-stick vegetable cooking spray. Pour tomato sauce over all. Bake at 375° until hot and bubbling.

COUNTS AS: 1 Lunch Protein List C
1 Vegetable List A Selection

▌ SALMON CROQUETTES ▌
125 calories

---

3 oz (⅓ cup) canned pink salmon

---

2 teaspoons dehydrated onion flakes

---

2 oz (¼ cup) finely diced celery

Dijon mustard to taste

Horseradish (optional)

Drain and flake salmon. Add onion flakes and celery, then enough mustard to moisten. Shape salmon mixture into patties, place on foil, and bake at 350° for 20 minutes, or until slightly browned. Serve with horseradish if desired.

COUNTS AS: 1 Dinner Protein List A

DAY 25 PLAIN

Breakfast

8 oz (½ medium) grapefruit

1 soft-boiled egg

¾ oz (¾ cup) cornflakes

2 tablespoons unprocessed bran

8 oz (1 cup) skim milk

Lunch

Large tossed salad

4 teaspoons low-calorie salad dressing

2–4 oz (¼–½ cup) water-packed tuna

1 oz (1 slice) rye bread

2 teaspoons imitation mayonnaise

Dinner

Large tossed salad

4 teaspoons low-calorie salad dressing

4–6 oz cooked Rock Cornish hen

4 oz (½ cup) cooked sliced asparagus

4 oz (½ cup) cooked sliced beets

Add to or between meals 1 Milk Selection (see page 176) and 1 Fruit Selection (see pages 177–78).

DAY 25 GOURMET

Breakfast

12 oz (½ small) cantaloupe

2 oz (¼ cup) low-fat cottage cheese

1 oz (¾ medium) bran muffin

1 teaspoon butter

Lunch

Large tossed salad

4 teaspoons low-calorie salad dressing

* Impossible Vegetable Quiche

6 oz (¾ cup) skim milk

Dinner

Large tossed salad

4 teaspoons low-calorie salad dressing

* Sweet and Sour Whitefish

Add to or between meals 1 Milk Selection (see page 176) and 1 Fruit Selection (see pages 177–78).

DAY 25 GOURMET
RECIPES

▮ IMPOSSIBLE VEGETABLE QUICHE ▮
(3 servings) 315 calories per serving

4 oz (½ cup) canned sliced mushrooms, drained
1 10-oz package frozen chopped broccoli, thawed
1 10-oz package frozen cauliflowerets, thawed and chopped
1 10-oz package frozen chopped spinach, thawed and well drained (all vegetables can be fresh)
8 oz (1 cup) part-skim ricotta cheese
2 eggs
6 tablespoons self-rising flour
6 oz (¾ cup) skim milk
Parsley, dry minced onions, salt, and pepper to taste

Mix together all vegetables and place in cake pan coated with no-stick vegetable cooking spray. Mix together remaining ingredients with hand mixer and pour over vegetables. Bake at 400° for 30–35 minutes.

EACH SERVING COUNTS AS: 1 Lunch Protein List C
1 Bread Selection
¼ Milk Selection

∎ SWEET AND SOUR WHITEFISH ∎
310 calories

4 oz (½ cup) sliced onion
8 oz (1 cup) water
2 oz (¼ cup) white vinegar
Artificial sweetener (to equal sweetness of 6 teaspoons sugar)
Dash of salt and pepper
¼ teaspoon ground ginger
6 oz raw whitefish

Place sliced onions in saucepan and add water. Simmer uncovered for 10 minutes. Add vinegar, artificial sweetener, salt, pepper, and ginger, and simmer for 5 minutes more. Turn off heat and add fish to saucepan mixture. Marinate for 10 minutes (if necessary, add more water to cover fish). Then simmer, covered, for ½ hour.

COUNTS AS: 1 Dinner Protein List A
1 Vegetable List A Selection

DAY 26 PLAIN

Breakfast

8 oz (1 medium) orange
1 oz lox
1 oz (½ medium) whole-wheat bagel
1 teaspoon cream cheese

Lunch

Large tossed salad
4 teaspoons low-calorie salad dressing

2–4 oz broiled chicken

4 oz (½ cup) cooked cauliflowerets

8 oz (1 cup) skim milk

Dinner

Large tossed salad

2 teaspoons low-calorie salad dressing

4–6 oz broiled veal burger

1 oz (½ medium) whole-grain roll

1 tablespoon ketchup

Add to or between meals 1 Milk Selection (see page 176) and 1 Fruit Selection (see pages 177–78).

DAY 26 GOURMET

Breakfast

* Pink Panther

Lunch

* Julie's Waldorf Salad

1 oz (½ medium) roll

Dinner

Large tossed salad

4 teaspoons low-calorie salad dressing

4–6 oz (½–¾ cup) canned minced clams

3 oz (⅓ cup) cooked spaghetti

4 oz (½ cup) home-style meatless oil-free tomato sauce

Add to or between meals 1 Milk Selection (see page 176).

DAY 26 GOURMET RECIPES

▮ PINK PANTHER ▮
240 calories

8 oz (1 cup) skim milk

1 oz (¼ cup) wheat germ

8 oz (1 cup) fresh strawberries

Artificial sweetener to taste

1 teaspoon vanilla extract

Ice cubes (as desired)

In blender, place milk, wheat germ, strawberries, sweetener, and vanilla, and blend on low until mixed. Add ice cubes one at a time, blending on high after each addition. Serve immediately.

COUNTS AS: 1 Breakfast Protein List D
                 1 Fruit Selection
                 1 Milk Selection
                 ⅓ Daily flavoring extract from Free Food List

▮ JULIE'S WALDORF SALAD ▮
425 calories

4 oz (½ cup) cubed cooked chicken
4 oz (1 medium) apple, unpeeled and cut into chunks
2 medium stalks celery, cut into chunks
2 teaspoons imitation mayonnaise
Chunks of lettuce (as desired)
Onion powder to taste
½ oz (1 tablespoon) chopped mixed nuts

Toss together all ingredients except nuts. Sprinkle salad with nuts.

COUNTS AS: 1 Lunch Protein List B
1 Fruit Selection
2 Oil and Condiment Selections

DAY 27 PLAIN

Breakfast

8 oz (½ medium) grapefruit
2 oz (¼ cup) low-fat cottage cheese
4 oz (½ cup) cooked oatmeal
2 tablespoons unprocessed bran
8 oz (1 cup) skim milk

Lunch

Large tossed salad
4 teaspoons low-calorie salad dressing

2–4 oz cooked white turkey meat

1 oz (1 slice) rye bread

2 teaspoons imitation mayonnaise

Dinner

Large tossed salad

4 teaspoons low-calorie salad dressing

4–6 oz baked Rock Cornish hen

Broccoli (as desired)

8 oz (1 cup) fresh strawberries

Add to or between meals 1 Milk Selection (see page 176).

DAY 27 GOURMET

Breakfast

* Blender Breakfast

1 oz (¾ small) corn muffin

Lunch

Large tossed salad

4 teaspoons low-calorie salad dressing

2 oz lean roast beef

1 oz (1 slice) rye bread

Dinner

* Artichoke-Spinach Salad

* East India Chicken

Add to or between meals 1 Milk Selection (see page 176) and ½ Fruit Selection (see pages 177–78).

DAY 27 GOURMET RECIPES

▮ BLENDER BREAKFAST ▮
240 calories

4 oz (½ medium) banana, weighed with peel

1 oz (¼ cup) wheat germ

8 oz (1 cup) skim milk

Artificial sweetener to taste

Peel banana, wrap in aluminum foil, and freeze for about 2–3 hours, or overnight. Then place all ingredients, including banana, in blender and blend at medium speed until mixed. Serve immediately.

COUNTS AS: 1 Breakfast Protein List D
1 Fruit Selection
1 Milk Selection

▮ ARTICHOKE-SPINACH SALAD ▮
190 calories

4 oz (8 whole) cold artichoke or palm hearts
4 oz (2 cups) chopped fresh spinach
4 oz (2 cups) lettuce leaves
4 oz (½ cup) sliced fresh mushrooms
4 oz (½ medium) cucumber, thinly sliced
¼ teaspoon dried tarragon
Sprinkling of parsley flakes
Salt and pepper to taste
2 teaspoons vegetable oil
Vinegar (as desired)

Toss together vegetables and seasonings. Serve topped with oil and vinegar.

COUNTS AS: 1 Vegetable List A Selection
2 Oil and Condiment Selections

▮ EAST INDIA CHICKEN ▮
(2 servings) 375 calories per serving

½ teaspoon saffron
1½ tablespoons boiling water
¼ teaspoon ground coriander
¼ teaspoon ground cumin
½ teaspoon chopped fresh ginger or ¼ teaspoon powdered ginger
⅛ teaspoon Tabasco sauce
1 clove garlic, minced
4 oz (½ cup) low-fat plain yogurt
14 oz boned and skinned chicken breasts (will cook down to 12 oz)
2 oz (¼ cup) freshly squeezed lemon juice
Salt to taste

Measure saffron into small bowl. Pour boiling water over it, and cool to room temperature. Add coriander, cumin, ginger, Tabasco, garlic, and yogurt; mix well. Brush chicken pieces with lemon juice, then sprinkle with salt. Coat with yogurt sauce and arrange in large glass dish or platter. Marinate chicken pieces in yogurt sauce in refrigerator for 12 hours, or overnight. Arrange pieces on rack in shallow roasting or broiler pan. Pour any remaining marinade over chicken. Roast at 400° for 15 minutes. Reduce heat to 350° and roast 30 minutes longer. Do not eat any of the pan drippings.

EACH SERVING COUNTS AS: 1 Dinner Protein List B
½ Milk Selection

DAY 28 PLAIN

Breakfast

8 oz (1 medium) orange

1 egg scrambled with 2 tablespoons unprocessed bran

8 oz (1 cup) low-calorie hot chocolate, made with artificial sweetener and skim milk

Lunch

Large tossed salad

4 teaspoons low-calorie salad dressing

2 oz (2 slices) liverwurst

2 oz (2 slices) whole-grain bread

8 oz (1 cup) skim milk

Dinner

Large tossed salad

4 teaspoons low-calorie salad dressing

6 oz cooked white turkey meat

2 oz (¼ small) baked sweet potato with

1 teaspoon butter

Add to or between meals 1 Fruit Selection (see pages 177–78).

DAY 28 GOURMET

Breakfast

4 oz (½ cup) orange juice

* 3 Pumpkin Muffins

1 teaspoon butter

Lunch

Large tossed salad

4 teaspoons low-calorie salad dressing

2–4 oz (¼–½ cup) cold cooked shrimp

8 oz (1 cup) tomato juice

Dinner

Large tossed salad

4 teaspoons low-calorie salad dressing

4–6 oz cooked white turkey meat

Broccoli (as desired)

* Yogurt Rice Pudding

Add with or between meals 1 Fruit Selection
(see pages 177–78).

DAY 28 GOURMET
RECIPES

▮ PUMPKIN MUFFINS ▮
(12 muffins, 4 servings)
255 calories per serving

2½ oz (1⅓ cups) 100% bran cereal
1⅓ cups nonfat dry milk
3 teaspoons baking powder
2 teaspoons pumpkin-pie spice
Artificial sweetener (to equal sweetness of 8 teaspoons sugar)
2 tablespoons unprocessed bran
12 oz (1½ cups) canned unsweetened pumpkin
4 eggs

Combine all dry ingredients. Add pumpkin and eggs, and mix until smooth. Let stand 5 minutes. Spoon into nonstick muffin tins or muffin tins coated with no-stick vegetable cooking spray. Bake at 375° for 20–25 minutes.

3 MUFFINS COUNT AS: 1 Breakfast Protein List C
1 Vegetable List A Selection
1 Bread Selection
1 Milk Selection

▮ YOGURT RICE PUDDING ▮
165 calories

4 oz (½ cup) low-fat plain yogurt
3 oz (⅓ cup) cooked enriched white rice
Artificial sweetener (to equal sweetness of 4 teaspoons sugar)
Ground cinnamon to taste

Combine all ingredients. Mix well and refrigerate.

COUNTS AS: 1 Bread Selection
1 Milk Selection

DAY 29 PLAIN

Breakfast

8 oz (½ medium) grapefruit
1 poached egg
1 oz (1 slice) whole-grain bread, toasted
8 oz (1 cup) skim milk

Lunch

Large tossed salad
4 teaspoons low-calorie salad dressing
2-4 (¼-½ cup) water-packed tuna
4 oz (1 medium) apple

Dinner

Large tossed salad
4 teaspoons low-calorie salad dressing

4–6 oz broiled swordfish

4 oz (½ cup) green peas with

1 teaspoon butter

Add to or between meals 1 Bread Selection (see page 175) and 1 Milk Selection (see page 176).

DAY 29 GOURMET

Breakfast

* Banana Omelet

1 oz (¾ small) corn muffin

8 oz (1 cup) skim milk

Lunch

Large tossed salad

4 teaspoons low-calorie salad dressing

* Stuffed Mushrooms

1 oz (½ medium) whole-grain roll

1 teaspoon butter

Dinner

Large tossed salad

4 teaspoons low-calorie salad dressing

4–6 oz cooked Rock Cornish hen

4 oz (½ cup) cooked sliced carrots

* Strawberry Rhubarb Dessert

Add to or between meals 1 Milk Selection (see page 176).

DAY 29 GOURMET
RECIPES

▮ BANANA OMELET ▮
130 calories

---

1 egg, well beaten

---

2 tablespoons water

---

4 oz (½ medium) banana, weighed with peel

Beat together egg and water. Peel and slice banana. Coat small frying pan with no-stick vegetable cooking spray. Heat pan for about 1 minute over medium heat, and then add egg. When egg is firm on all sides, place banana slices on top and fold egg over it. Cook until set.

COUNTS AS: 1 Breakfast Protein List C
1 Fruit Selection

▮ STUFFED MUSHROOMS ▮
70 calories

---

4 oz (6 large) fresh whole mushrooms

---

4 oz (½ cup) low-fat cottage cheese

Onion flakes and parsley flakes to taste

Dash of pepper

Remove and chop mushroom stems (reserve the mushroom caps) and add to remaining ingredients in bowl. Mix together. Stuff mushroom caps with cheese mixture. Bake at 375° for 25 minutes in nonstick pan or pan coated with no-stick vegetable cooking spray.

COUNTS AS: 1 Lunch Protein List C

▮ STRAWBERRY RHUBARB DESSERT ▮
85 calories

---

2 envelopes unflavored gelatin

---

12 oz (1½ cups) sugar-free diet strawberry soda

Artificial sweetener (to equal sweetness of 6 teaspoons sugar)

---

8 oz (1 cup) precooked unsweetened rhubarb, heated

---

8 oz (1 cup) fresh whole strawberries

Place gelatin in mold dish and moisten with 4 oz (½ cup) soda. In saucepan, bring remaining soda to boiling and add it and sweetener to gelatin, stirring until dissolved. Add hot rhubarb and strawberries. Mix and refrigerate.

COUNTS AS: 1 Fruit Selection

DAY 30 PLAIN

Breakfast

---

8 oz (½ medium) grapefruit

½ oz (1 teaspoon) chopped mixed nuts

¾ oz (¾ cup) cornflakes

---

2 tablespoons unprocessed bran

---

8 oz (1 cup) skim milk

Lunch

Large spinach salad

---

4 teaspoons low-calorie salad dressing

2–4 oz broiled chicken

8 oz (1 cup) fresh strawberries with

4 teaspoons sour cream

Dinner

Large tossed salad

4 teaspoons low-calorie salad dressing

4–6 oz broiled filet of sole

3 oz (⅓ cup) enriched white rice

4 oz (½ small) cooked butternut squash

Add to or between meals 1 Milk Selection (see page 176).

DAY 30 GOURMET

Breakfast

1 soft-boiled egg

8 oz (1 cup) low-calorie hot chocolate

1 oz (1 slice) whole-wheat bread

Lunch

* Spinach Parmesan

8 oz (1 cup) fresh strawberries with

4 teaspoons sour cream

Dinner

Large spinach salad

4 teaspoons low-calorie salad dressing

Polynesian Chicken Kabobs

3 oz (⅓ cup) cooked brown rice with

1 teaspoon butter

Add to or between meals 1 Milk Selection (see page 176).

DAY 30 GOURMET RECIPES

▮ SPINACH PARMESAN ▮
250 calories

4 oz (1 cup) cooked spinach, drained and chopped

Salt and pepper to taste

⅛ teaspoon ground nutmeg

1 egg, slightly beaten

1 oz (2 tablespoons) grated Parmesan cheese

Place spinach in saucepan. Season with salt, pepper, and nutmeg. Add egg and grated cheese. Mix well. Cook, stirring, over very low heat for 2–3 minutes, or until egg is set.

COUNTS AS: 1 Lunch Protein List C

▮ POLYNESIAN CHICKEN KABOBS ▮
440 calories

1 oz (⅛ cup) unsweetened pineapple juice from unsweetened canned chunk-style pineapple
1 tablespoon soy sauce
½ teaspoon powdered ginger
Onion flakes, salt, and pepper to taste
7 oz (⅞ cup) chicken cubes (will cook down to 6 oz)
8 oz (1 large can) button mushrooms
4 oz (1 large) green pepper, cut into squares
3 oz (⅓ cup) canned unsweetened chunk-style pineapple

In bowl, mix pineapple juice, soy sauce, ginger, onion flakes, salt, and pepper. Add remaining ingredients, cover, and marinate in refrigerator for several hours, preferably overnight, mixing occasionally. Then alternately skewer pieces. Broil or barbecue until chicken is browned.

COUNTS AS: 1 Dinner Protein List B
1 Fruit Selection
1 Daily soy sauce from Free Food List

Note: This recipe is ideal for summer picnics.

9. SETTING UP YOUR OWN ONE MONTH LIGHTER PROGRAM

Now that you have completed the One Month Lighter Program, you've lost some weight and you've learned quite a bit about us and yourself and how to control food intake. Now it is time for you to set up your own One Month Lighter Program.

Why "One Month"? Because one month isn't a very long time. It is an attainable goal. One reason many people give up on their diets is because it seems like an endless task. We at Lean Line often repeat the story of the pendulum that Dwight Lyman Moody, the nineteenth-century evangelist and founder of the Northfield and Mount Hermon schools in Massachusetts, used to tell.

Once there was a pendulum sitting in a clock shop, waiting to be put on a new clock. It began to think about how long it would have to work before the big wheels wore out and its work would be done. It would be expected to tick night and day, so many times per minute, 60 times that every hour, 24 times that every day, 365 times that every year—millions of ticks.

"I can never do it," said the pendulum.

But the old clockmaker said, "Can you do one tick at a time?"

"Oh, yes," said the pendulum. "I can do that."

"Well, that's all that is required of you."

So the pendulum went to work, one tick at a time, and is ticking yet, quite cheerfully.

If you start thinking about all the weight you want to lose, you may be overwhelmed. Instead, take it one day at a time for just one month, as you did with the progam we designed for you.

You can be creative about your program and add your own personal touches. All good things to eat are not fattening. Many tempting flavors can be added to vegetables, meats, salads, and eggs without hiking the caloric value.

Bouillon, lemon, orange juice, grated rinds, vinegars, herbs, and spices are of little or no caloric value, for example, but can add gourmet flavor to foods. Experiment.

We strongly advise you to continue broiling or roasting your meats, fish, and poultry, as you did in our One Month Lighter Program. You can rub meats with unusual seasonings and flavorings, adding deliciously subtle flavors. For beef or lamb, use basil, rosemary, garlic powder, or dry mustard. The flavor of veal, chicken, and fish is enhanced remarkably by rosemary and savory.

Vegetables are especially important to any sound plan for dieting, so become an expert in combining them with herbs to achieve new and delightful flavors.

Cook fresh-cut green beans in a small amount of boiling water, for instance, to which ½ teaspoon of dried savory has been added. Serve with a spoonful of tomato juice and chopped parsley or basil.

Simmer fresh or frozen brussels sprouts until barely tender in a small amount of boiling salted water to which a dash of thyme has been added. Drain and serve with a sprinkling of sweet marjoram and chopped parsley.

Shred cabbage and cook, covered, in a little water to which a few caraway seeds have been added, along with a dash of marjoram, savory, or dill weed. Serve with some crushed marjoram.

For delicate flavor, cook fresh or frozen peas in a small amount of beef bouillon until tender and the liquid has been absorbed.

Other good flavor combinations are fresh spinach with nutmeg, paprika, rosemary, chives, or marjoram; corn with mustard or thyme; zucchini squash with thyme, nutmeg, or Worcestershire sauce; carrots with ginger, thyme, or nutmeg; and eggs with basil or chervil.

All right, now you are ready to use your creativity to set up your program.

You should plan menus a week in advance and keep a careful record of everything you eat and your feelings while eating (see Food and Emotions Chart on page 74).

We urge you to continue weighing yourself only once a week, as you were asked to do during our One Month Lighter Program. If you do it more often, it can be distracting and discouraging, since your weight can vary slightly from day to day depending on water retention. It is the total weekly loss that counts. Incidentally, if you have a tendency to retain a lot of water, you should avoid sauerkraut, pickles, bouillon, diet soda, and saccharin. All of these are normally high in salt and thus cause fluid retention.

Remember, a Lean Line Program is balanced nutritionally. There are six basic food lists from which you will be selecting your food intake for each day. These are the Protein, Vegetable, Bread, and Milk, Fruit, Oil and Condiment lists. We have also provided two Bonus Lists.

PROTEIN

One protein selection at each meal is a requirement. There are three meals every day: breakfast, lunch, and dinner. There is no such meal as brunch.

There are four lists of protein from which you will select your quota of protein for each day. Check the top of each list carefully for the correct portion of protein that you should eat at breakfast, lunch, and dinner.

Protein selections should be varied constantly to assure maximum weight loss and nutrition.

We suggest you cook protein before weighing or measuring it. The weights listed refer to meats that have been boned, skinned, and cooked.

Limit hard cheese to 4 oz (four slices) per week, since it is high in fat. However, to round out your program and for your enjoyment, it is acceptable. A hard cheese is anything that you can slice, such as Swiss, cheddar, and mozzarella.

Limit your intake of eggs to five or less a week, since current medical opinion is that eggs contribute greatly to high blood cholesterol.

Protein List A
Trimmed Weights, Cooked

1 oz = 1 Breakfast Selection
2 oz = 1 Lunch Selection
3 oz = 1 Dinner Selection for women
4 oz = 1 Dinner Selection for men and preteens

Anchovies
Beef, lean
Halibut
Ham, baked or boiled
Herring
Hot dogs, all-beef, chicken,
    or turkey
Lamb
Liver
Liverwurst
Lox
Mackerel

Pheasant
Pork, roast or chops
Rabbit
Salmon
Sardines, water-packed
Shad
Tongue
Tripe
Tuna, oil-packed
Turkey, dark meat
Whitefish

Protein List B
Trimmed Weights, Cooked

2 oz = 1 Breakfast Selection
2–4 oz = 1 Lunch Selection
4–6 oz = 1 Dinner Selection for women
6–8 oz = 1 Dinner Selection for men and preteens

Bass
Bluefish
Chicken
Chicken roll
Clams
Cod
Crab meat
Flounder
Fluke
Frogs legs
Haddock
Lobster
Oysters

Red snapper
Rock Cornish hen
Scallops
Shrimp
Sole
Swordfish
Trout
Tuna, water-packed or fresh
Turbot
Turkey, white meat
Turkey ham
Turkey pastrami
Turkey roll

Veal   Veal sausage, Lean Line
Veal franks, Lean Line   brand only
   brand only   Venison

Protein List C

BREAKFAST

Cheese, cottage	2 oz (¼ cup)
Cheese, farmer	2 oz (¼ cup)
Cheese, hard	1 oz (1 slice), limit 4 oz (4 slices) per week
Cheese, pot	2 oz (¼ cup)
Eggs	1, limit 5 per week
Egg substitute	1½ oz (3 tablespoons), liquid measure
Ricotta, part-skim	2 oz (¼ cup)

LUNCH

Cheese, cottage	4 oz (½ cup)
Cheese, farmer	4 oz (½ cup)
Cheese, hard	2 oz (2 slices), limit 4 oz (4 slices) per week
Cheese, pot	4 oz (½ cup)
Eggs	2, limit 5 per week
Egg substitute	3 oz (6 tablespoons), liquid measure
Ricotta, part-skim	4 oz (½ cup)

DINNER

Cheese, cottage	4–6 oz (½–¾ cup)
Cheese, farmer	4–6 oz (½–¾ cup)
Cheese, hard	3 oz (3 slices), limit 4 oz (4 slices) per week
Cheese, pot	4–6 oz (½–¾ cup)
Eggs	3, limit 5 per week
Egg substitute	4½ oz (9 tablespoons), liquid measure
Ricotta, part-skim	4–6 oz (½–¾ cup)

Protein List D

BEANS, LENTILS, PEAS, SOYBEANS, TOFU, SOYBEAN CURD (COOKED WEIGHT)

2 oz (¼ cup)	*= 1 Breakfast Selection*
2–4 oz (¼–½ cup)	*= 1 Lunch Selection*
4–6 oz (½–¾ cup)	*= 1 Dinner Selection*

WHEAT GERM

1 oz (¼ cup)	*= 1 Breakfast Selection*
2 oz (½ cup)	*= 1 Lunch Selection*
3 oz (1 cup)	*= 1 Dinner Selection*

NUTS, PEANUT BUTTER, SESAME SEEDS, TOASTED SOYBEANS

½ oz (1 tablespoon)	*= 1 Breakfast Selection*
1 oz (2 tablespoons)	*= 1 Lunch Selection*
1½ oz (3 tablespoons)	*= 1 Dinner Selection*

Note: Eat the equivalent of only one protein selection at each meal. All protein selections may be mixed and matched. For example, a 2-oz protein lunch selection may include 1 oz ham from List A and 1 oz Swiss cheese from List C.

VEGETABLES

Vegetables are of the utmost importance to your nutritionally balanced weight-control program. There is increasing evidence that they not only serve as sources of nutrients and fiber, they protect against cancer, heart disease, and lowered immunity in general.

Select from either Vegetable Lists A, B, or C at least once daily. List B may be used up to three times a week in place of List A if you wish. On a given day, if you do not choose a vegetable from List A or B, then one from List C—minimum of 4 oz (½ cup)—becomes required. Vegetables from List C, used freely without weighing or measuring, may be eaten along with those from List A or List B. However, remember that a vegetable from List A and one from List B should not be eaten together on the same day. Check the top of each list carefully for the correct amount.

Fresh vegetables are preferable. If they are not available, then frozen is preferred over canned, although canned vegetables (low-salt if available) are still preferable to no vegetables at all.

Beans, peas, and lentils may be used either as vegetables (List B) or as protein (List D) and must be accurately measured accordingly.

Vegetable List A

4 oz (½ cup) = 1 Selection

Artichoke hearts   Beets
Bamboo shoots   Brussels sprouts

Carrots, cooked or raw
Collards
Dandelion greens
Kohlrabi
Leeks
Okra

Onions, weighed raw
Pumpkin
Snow peas
Tomato sauce or purée
Turnips
Winter squash

Vegetable List B

You may select from this list up to three times a week in place of List A if you wish.

2 oz (¼ cup) cooked = 1 Selection

Baked beans, without pork
Beans (kidney and others)
Lentils
Lima Beans

Sweet potato
Tomato paste
Yams

4 oz (½ cup) cooked = 1 Selection

Corn, whole-kernel (or 6 oz
   cob, 6 x 2 in.)
Parsnips

Peas, green
Potatoes
Water chestnuts

Vegetable List C

With the exception of tomatoes, you may choose from this list freely without weighing or measuring. If you do not choose a vegetable from List A or B, then a vegetable from List C—a minimum of 4 oz (½ cup)—is required.

Asparagus
Beet greens
Broccoli

Cabbage
Cauliflower
Celery

Chives
Chicory
Cucumbers
Eggplant
Endive
Escarole
Green beans, including
    wax beans, French-style
    or regular
Kale
Lettuce
Mushrooms
Mustard greens
Parsley
Peppers, red and green
Pickles, dill
Pimentos, water-packed

Radishes
Rhubarb
Sauerkraut
Spinach
Sprouts, all varieties
Spaghetti squash
Summer squash, yellow
    and zucchini
Swiss chard
Tomatoes, cooked or
    canned, limit 8 oz (1
    cup) daily
Tomatoes, fresh, limit 8 oz
    (1 cup) daily
Tomatoes, sour
Turnip greens
Watercress

BREAD

As Dr. Fisher, our nutrition consultant, says, people may get sick of sweets, but they never get tired of eating breads. They are common to most of the world's dinner tables, and we include them in our program. It's the amount that counts. One easy trick we found is that if you love hard rolls like we do, pull out the inside of the roll and leave the crust. Then you can stuff the roll with a salad or meat and have a "big" sandwich without the "big" calories.

Women should choose two bread selections daily, and men and preteens, three selections daily.

Bread Selections

Bagels	1 oz (½ small, 3 in. diam.)
Bran muffins	1 oz (¾ medium, 3 in. diam.)
Bread or rolls, plain (packaged, bakery, or homemade)	1 oz (1 slice or ½ medium roll)
Breadsticks	¾ oz (7–8 small or 2–3 large sticks)
Bread crumbs, plain (commercial)	½ oz (2 tablespoons)
Cereal, cooked	4 oz (½ cup)
Cereal, dry (puffed, flaked, or shredded—not sugar-coated)	¾ oz (¾ cup)
Cornbread or corn muffins	1 oz (¾ small, 2½ in. diam.)
English muffin	1 oz (½ medium, 4½ in. diam.)
Flour, cornstarch, or arrowroot	2 tablespoons
Matzo	¾ oz (¾ sheet)
Matzo meal	¾ oz (3 tablespoons)
Melba toast, plain	½ oz (7 pieces)
Pancakes	1 oz (4 in. diam.) cooked
Pita bread	1 oz (1 small or ½ large)
Rice	3 oz (⅓ cup) cooked
Rice cakes	2 cakes
Spaghetti or noodles	3 oz (⅓ cup) cooked
Tapioca	2 tablespoons uncooked
Tortillas	1 oz (7 in. diam.)
Waffles	1 oz (4 in. diam.) cooked

MILK

Milk is an excellent source of calcium, and there is increasing evidence that many of us don't get enough to prevent bone deterioration in later years or to combat heart irregularities. You should choose two selections daily.

Milk Selections

Everyone must choose 2 selections daily. Measurements referred to on this list are liquid *measurements.*

Buttermilk	6 oz (¾ cup)
Evaporated skim milk	4 oz (½ cup)
Fat-free milk, 1% fat or less	8 oz (1 cup)
Nonfat dry milk, reconstituted	8 oz (1 cup)
Skim milk	8 oz (1 cup)
Yogurt, low-fat plain	4 oz (½ cup)

Weights listed below are scale *weighed. (See Bonus List B for ice cream.)*

Frozen dietary dessert	2½ oz (⅓ cup)
Frozen low-fat yogurt	2 oz (¼ cup)
Frozen yogurt bar, uncoated	1 bar

FRUITS

Fruits are a treat and add not only sweetness and color to any diet but provide vitamins and fiber. Women on the Lean Line Program should choose two selections daily, and men and preteens, three selections daily. One of these selections must be a fruit high in vitamin C. An asterisk (*) indicates that the fruit is high in vitamin C.

The weight of fruits includes pits, peel, or skin wherever applicable.

Use fresh, frozen, or canned fruit packed in unsweetened juice or water. The juice is measured separately.

Never use fruit that has added sugar. Of course, whole fresh fruit is preferable to canned and frozen, but the latter will do when fresh fruit is not available.

Fruit Selections

4 oz = 1 Selection (scale weighed)

Apples	1 small or ½ medium
Applesauce, unsweetened	½ cup
Apricots	2 medium
Bananas	½ medium
Blackberries	½ cup
Blueberries	½ cup
Cherries	½ cup
Cranberries	1 cup
*Grapefruit sections, unsweetened	½ cup
Grapes	½ cup
Mangoes	½ medium
Melon balls, unsweetened	½ cup
Nectarines	2 medium
*Orange sections, unsweetened	½ cup
*Papaya	⅓ medium
Peaches	1 medium
Pears	1 small
Pineapple sections, unsweetened	½ cup

Plums	2 medium
Raspberries	⅔ cup

8 oz = 1 Selection (scale weighed)

*Grapefruits	½ medium
*Oranges	1 medium
*Strawberries	1 cup
*Tangerines	1 large

12 oz (½ small or ¼ medium) = 1 Selection (scale weighed with peel or rind)

Melons, all

Any of the following = 1 Selection as indicated (scale weighed)

All dried fruits (raisins, figs, dates, etc.)	½ oz (1 tablespoon)
Prunes	1 oz (⅛ cup, or 5 small/medium prunes)

Juice 2 oz (¼ cup) = 1 Selection (measured in measuring cup)

Cranberry	Prune

Juice 4 oz (½ cup) = 1 Selection (measured in measuring cup)

Apple juice or cider	*Orange
Grape	*Papaya
*Grapefruit	Pineapple
Low-calorie cranberry	*Tangerine
Nectars, all	

OILS AND CONDIMENTS

Oils and condiments give our food pizzaz. As we promised at the beginning of this book, food doesn't have to be dull and tasteless to be nonfattening. You must choose three selections of the following daily.

Oil and Condiment Selections

Avocado	4 teaspoons
Bacon, baked or broiled on rack	1 strip
Butter	1 teaspoon
Butter, whipped	1½ teaspoons
Chili sauce	2 tablespoons
Cocoa unsweetened	1 tablespoon
Cream cheese	1 teaspoon
Cream cheese, imitation or whipped	1½ teaspoons
Fat or oil	1 teaspoon
Gravy or sauce	2 teaspoons
Heavy cream, not whipped	1 teaspoon
Heavy cream, whipped	1 tablespoon
Heavy cream, imitation—whipped	1½ tablespoon
Ketchup	2 tablespoons
Margarine	1 teaspoon
Margarine, diet	2 teaspoons
Mayonnaise	1 teaspoon
Mayonnaise, imitation	2 teaspoons
Nuts, chopped	1 tablespoon
Olives, green or black	5 small
Peanut Butter	1 teaspoon
Salad dressing	2 teaspoons
Salad dressing, diet or low calorie	4 teaspoons
Sour cream	4 teaspoons

BONUS FOODS

If you have utilized all foods on the program and you are still hungry or are a confirmed snacker, you may choose one of the following selections daily. (It is not required that you choose a selection from Bonus List A.)

Bonus List A

1 oz from Protein List A
or
2 oz from Protein list B
or
1 Protein List C Selection—
breakfast portion
or
1 Protein-List D Selection—
breakfast portion
or

Vegetable List A or B Selection
or
1 Bread Selection
or
1 Milk Selection
or
1 Fruit Selection
or
1 Oil and Condiment Selection

Bonus List B

May be chosen three times a week in place of Bonus List A after the fourth dieting week

Beer	8 oz (¾ cup)
Cake, plain, without icing or lumps	¾ oz (⅓ slice, 3 x 3 x 1 in.)
Carbonated beverages, containing sugar	8 oz (¾ cup)
Cookies, plain, without lumps	¾ oz (2 small/medium pieces)
Crackers, plain	¾ oz (6–7 small or 3–4 medium pieces)
Cranberry sauce	3 tablespoons
Cupcake, plain, without icing or lumps	¾ oz (½ medium, 2¾ in. diam.)

Doughnut, plain, without
    icing or lumps   ¾ oz (¾ medium)
Honey   4 teaspoons
Ice cream, plain, without
    nuts or chips (vanilla,
    chocolate, strawberry,
    peach, coffee)   ½ cup
Liquor (brandy, gin, rye,
    scotch, or vodka)   1 oz (⅛ cup)
Marmalade, jelly, or jam   5 teaspoons
Popcorn   1 oz (5 cups)
Pretzels   1 oz (2 rods, 5 thin-twisted
                             pieces, or 50 thin sticks,
                             3⅛ in.)

Salami, bologna, or corned
    beef, lean   ¾ oz (1 very thin slice)
Sherbet   ½ cup
Shredded coconut   3 tablespoons
Soups (canned, bottled, or
    dried)   8 oz (1 cup)
    Borscht   Tomato
    Chicken with noodles   Turkey with noodles
    Chicken with rice   Vegetable
    Clam chowder (Manhat-
    tan)
Sugar, white or brown   4 teaspoons
Syrup   4 teaspoons
Wines and Vermouth
    Dry   3 oz (⅓ cup)
    Sweet   1½ oz (⅛ cup, or 3 table-
                           spoons)

FREE FOODS

Free foods may be used whenever you wish, but they are not
required.

Please note that lemon and lime juices are fresh or frozen, not reconstituted. Any gelatin commercially prepared and flavored may be used, provided the label specifically reads "no sugar added," and no form of sugar (corn syrup, glucose, fructose, sucrose) is listed in ingredients.

Coffee, tea, and many cola-flavored diet sodas contain caffeine, which is an appetite stimulant. Be extremely cautious of these. Whenever possible, substitute decaffeinated coffees, noncola or caffeine-free diet soda, and the like.

Limit the intake of all diet soda to 24 oz (two 12-oz cans) per day because of the high sodium content. Water is still your best drink.

Free Food List

Artificial sweetener
Bouillon
Bran, unprocessed, 2 tablespoons per day
Coffee, preferably decaffeinated
Club soda or seltzer
Diet soda, sugar-free and caffeine-free, limit 24 oz or 2 12-oz cans per day
Extracts (vanilla, rum, etc.), up to 1 tablespoon per day
Gelatin, sugar-free, flavored
Gelatin, unflavored
Gum, plain, 5 sticks daily, regular or sugar-free
Horseradish
Juices, clam, clamato, tomato, vegetable, 8 oz (1 cup) per day
Lemon juice, fresh
Lime juice, fresh
Mustard
Sauces, soy, steak, or Worcestershire, 1 tablespoon per day
Seasonings, herbs, and spices
Tea
Vinegar

What about counting calories?

Dr. Arnold Lazarus maintains that counting calories is one of the best behavioral deterrents to overeating. It reinforces your control over your food intake.

But if despite everything—calorie counting, behavioral techniques, and choosing delicious, sensible selections—you still find yourself overeating, go through the BASIC ID again to find out what is going on inside. We've included a chart (page 74) to make it easy for you.

"Ask yourself," Dr. Lazarus advises, "what feelings am I experiencing? What unpleasant emotions? What can I do about them? Shall I practice relaxation? Shall I do some ex-

The following is a quick checklist indicating the number of selections of foods to be had daily on the program

FOOD	WOMEN			MEN AND PRETEENS		
	BREAKFAST	LUNCH	DINNER	BREAKFAST	LUNCH	DINNER
Protein	List A 1 oz or List B 2 oz or List C Breakfast Selection or List D Breakfast Selection	List A 2 oz or List B 2-4 oz or List C Lunch Selection or List D Lunch Selection	List A 3 oz or List B 4-6 oz or List C Dinner Selection or List D Dinner Selection	List A 1 oz or List B 2 oz or List C Breakfast Selection or List D Breakfast Selection	List A 2 oz or List B 2-4 oz or List C Lunch Selection or List D Lunch Selection	List A 4 oz or List B 6-8 oz or List C Dinner Selection or List D Dinner Selection
Vegetable	1 daily			1 daily		
Bread	2 daily			3 daily		
Milk	2 daily			2 daily		
Fruit	2 daily			3 daily		
Oil and Condiments	3 daily			3 daily		
Bonus	1 daily	(optional)		1 daily	(optional)	
Free Food		optional				

ercise? Shall I take longer walks? Am I not picturing myself in a positive light? Am I seeing myself in my mind not coping?"

Dr. Lazarus says he wants to get this message across to you because he feels it is of utmost importance: "If you go to a wedding or some other event where you eat a lot and then come home and feel like giving up, I say to you, 'You have not caused irreversible damage. For the next three or four or five days, be especially vigilant and carry on. Don't give up because you've had a slip up. Because you have had a tremendous binge should not discourage you from going back.'"

Since Lean Line is concerned with nutrition as well as controlled calories, we have included the following information that will help you look good both on the inside and the outside.

VITAMIN DEFICIENCY CAN HURT MORE THAN YOUR LOOKS

Vitamin deficiency can cause serious health problems. Vitamins are organic compounds found in small quantities in all kinds of foods. Each serves a specialized purpose in bodily functions. They are absolutely necessary for good health, growth, and maintenance.

Vitamins A, D, E, and K are known as the fat-soluble vitamins, since they do not dissolve in water.

The B vitamins and C are water-soluble vitamins. They may lose some of their potency in cooking, but generally not enough to worry about. To be on the safe side, however, always use small amounts of water when cooking fresh produce. Do not store fruits and vegetables for too long or overcook them. That can make them less potent, too.

Dietary allowances for vitamins are only approximations. Your own personal needs depend on age, sex, and lifestyle. A well-varied diet will provide all the necessary vitamins you need for good health.

FAT-SOLUBLE VITAMINS

Vitamin A is necessary for good eyesight and eyes that adapt readily to changes from light to dark, skeletal growth, and normal tooth structure. It is also necessary for the health of the mucous membranes lining the nose, throat, and other air passages. It can be stored in the body in the liver. Recommended daily allowance is 5,000 International Units.

FOODS HIGH IN VITAMIN A

The lists below are from highest in the vitamin to the lowest.

PROTEINS FROM PROTEIN LIST A.
Liver, Liverwurst

PROTEINS FROM PROTEIN LIST B.
Crab Meat, Swordfish, Chicken, Cornish Hen

VEGETABLES FROM VEGETABLE LIST A.
Pumpkin, Dandelion Greens, Carrots, Winter Squash, Collard Greens, Tomato Sauce

VEGETABLES FROM VEGETABLE LIST B.
Sweet Potato

VEGETABLES FROM VEGETABLE LIST C.
Spinach, Turnip Greens, Beet Greens, Kale, Swiss Chard, Mustard Greens, Parsley, Watercress, Broccoli, Pimentos (water-packed), Endive, Peppers (red)

FRUITS.
Mango, Apricots, Papaya, Melon, Cantaloupe, Nectarine

FREE FOODS.
Tomato Juice, Vegetable Juice

Vitamin D prevents rickets amd promotes normal bone growth. Daily recommended allowance for children is 400 International Units. Vitamin D can be stored in the body in the liver and can be formed from fatty material in the skin by ultraviolet light as in sunlight. It is found in a limited number of foods including fish-liver oils, vitamin D fortified foods including milk products.

Vitamin E is essential for the protection of the body cells from disintegrative changes. Good food sources include wheat and corn germ and most seed oils. It is found in moderate amounts in cereals, egg yolk, legumes, nuts and leafy vegetables.

Vitamin K is necessary in the formation of prothrombin which is vital to the proper clotting of blood. The adult daily requirement is as yet unknown. Food sources include cabbage, cauliflower, spinach, and other leafy vegetables, pork liver, soybean oil and other vegetable oils.

WATER-SOLUBLE VITAMINS

Vitamin C, or ascorbic acid, is necessary in the prevention of scurvy leading to sores in the mouth, swollen gums, hemorrhages, bone fragility, weakened capillary walls, and muscle weakness. Adult daily recommended level is 70 mg. for women and 75 mg. for men. To ameliorate the effects of common colds, 200 mg. per day has been recommended.

FOODS HIGH IN VITAMIN C

PROTEINS FROM PROTEIN LIST A.
Liver

PROTEINS FROM PROTEIN LIST D.
Peas

VEGETABLES FROM VEGETABLE LIST A.
Collard Greens, Dandelion Greens, Brussels Sprouts, Tomato Sauce, Tomatoes (canned), Turnips, Okra, Pea Pods

VEGETABLES FROM VEGETABLE LIST B.
Green Peas, Potatoes (white)

VEGETABLES FROM VEGETABLE LIST C.
Turnip Greens, Mustard Greens, Peppers (red), Bean Sprouts, Kale, Parsley, Peppers (green), Beet Greens, Broccoli, Pimentos (water-packed), Spinach, Asparagus, Cabbage, Watercress, Tomatoes (fresh), Sauerkraut, Swiss Chard, Zucchini, Radishes, Cauliflower, Green Beans

FRUITS.
Strawberries, Papaya, Grapefruit, Orange Sections, Mango, Raspberries, Tangerines, Pineapple, Blueberries, Nectarines

JUICES (NOT FORTIFIED).
Orange, Grapefruit, Tangerine

OILS AND CONDIMENTS.
Chili Sauce

FREE FOODS.
Tomato Juice, Vegetable Juice, Horseradish (raw)

Thiamine, or vitamin B_1, is necessary to prevent beriberi (a disease affecting the nerves and digestive system), fatigue, constipation. The adult human daily requirement is 0.8 to 1.2 mg. for women and 0.9 mg. to 1.2 for men.

FOODS HIGH IN VITAMIN B_1

PROTEINS FROM PROTEIN LIST A.
Pork (chops)

PROTEINS FROM PROTEIN LIST D.
Peas

Riboflavin, or vitamin B_2, is necessary for proper utilization of carbohydrates and amino acids in the body. Adult daily allowance is 1.2 to 1.8 mg. for women and 1.3 to 1.7 mg. for men.

FOODS HIGH IN VITAMIN B_2

PROTEINS FROM PROTEIN LIST A.
Liverwurst, Liver, Venison

PROTEINS FROM PROTEIN LIST B.
Veal, Oysters, Chicken

MILK
Nonfat dry milk

Niacin, or niacinamide or nicotinic acid (related compounds) is necessary in the prevention of pellagra (a disease involving the nerves and skin), and is an essential part of carbohydrate and amino acid metabolism. Adult daily allowance is 13 to 20 mg. for women and 15 to 19 mg. for men.

FOODS HIGH IN NIACIN

PROTEINS FROM PROTEIN LIST A.
Tuna, Shad, Rabbit, Halibut, Mackerel, Lox, Salmon, Venison, Liverwurst, Sardines, Lamb, Pork (chops), Liver

PROTEINS FROM PROTEIN LIST B.
Tuna, Turkey (white), Turkey Roll, Swordfish, Cornish Hen, Chicken, Veal, Haddock, Crab Meat, Oysters, Cod

PROTEINS FROM PROTEIN LIST D.
Peanuts, Roasted Nuts, Sesame Seeds

FREE FOODS.
Coffee (regular)

Pantothenic acid serves as a catalyst in the utilization of fats, sugars, and amino acids. No adult requirement has been established. (It is found in liver, organ meats, eggs, peanuts, legumes, mushrooms, salmon, yeast, wheat germ, and whole grains).

Vitamin B_6 or pyridoxine, pyridoxal, or pyridoxamine, is necessary for nerve function and to the proper metabolism of amino acids. Adult daily allowance is 1.5 to 2.0 mg. It is found in liver, pork, organ meats, legumes, seeds, grains, leafy foods, and potatoes.

Biotin is necessary for cell respiration. It is found in organ meats, egg yolks, milk, fruits, and leafy vegetables. Deficiencies are extremely rare and almost unknown in man.

Folacin and *vitamin B_{12}* are necessary for blood cell formation and prevention of anemia. Folacin is found in most leafy vegetables. B_{12} is closely related to nerve function and is found in organ meats, milk, eggs and fish. It is never found in vegetables or fruit and vegetarians are well advised to take some vitamin B_{12} supplement.

FIBER

Fiber in the diet plays an important role in laxation, in controlling the absorption of fats from the digestive tract and insuring proper movement of the digestive tract. The latter is very important in preventing the lodging of food in the folds of the intestine which could give rise to the production of toxic or irritating substances by bacteria. These, in turn, could cause difficulties or even cancer of the colon. Fruit, vegetables and whole grain cereal are good sources of fiber.

MINERALS

Approximately twenty-one mineral elements are now believed to be essential for human health. Most of these are required in only trace amounts. Their role, for the most part, is to help regulate metabolism. A few elements are needed for structural purposes, such as calcium and phosphorous. Several others are components of organic compounds, such as iron in hemoglobin, or cobalt in Vitamin B.

CALCIUM
Sardines, Yogurt, Almonds, Milk, Cheddar Cheese, Cottage Cheese, Broccoli, Turnip Greens

PHOSPHOROUS
Cheddar Cheese, Peanuts, Cottage Cheese, Halibut, Cod, Eggs, Pear, Bread, Lima Beans, Oatmeal

POTASSIUM
Dried Apricots, Avocado, Salmon, Chicken, Potato, Beef, Carrots, Banana, Tomato, Broccoli, Milk, Orange, Grapefruit, Apple, Liver

LOW SODIUM
Pineapple, Apple, Asparagus, Grapefruit, Broccoli, Raisins, Carrots, Sweet Potato

MAGNESIUM
Whole Grains, Peanuts, Spinach (raw), Soybeans

IRON
Dried Apricots, Beef, Lima Beans, Raisins, Enriched Bread, Spinach, Egg, Liver

10. YOUR NEW BEGINNING

What next? You've followed the One Month Lighter Program we designed for you and you've created your own One Month Lighter Program. What next? You should, after two months, have learned a new way to eat and to be thin.

We hope you can picture yourself as a thin person. One of the most difficult obstacles to overcome in weight reduction isn't getting rid of your fat body, it's getting rid of the fat that occupies your head. No matter how much weight you lose, if you still think of yourself as fat, if you look at your thinner body as just being temporary, it might become just that and you'll go back to your old habits, only to try yet another diet at some future date.

We suggest that if you want to avoid carrying around that

fat mental self-image, throw away your old, big-sized clothes. If you hang on to them, then you tell yourself that your new thinness is only a temporary state. Give your old clothes to charity. That way, you'll convince yourself you won't need them anymore. The more you act like a thin person, the greater your chance of being one.

It is now time for you to declare independence. You should be able to answer YES to all of the following:

- I now recognize the difference between tired and hungry and have learned to eat only when what I feel is real hunger.
- I've de-emphasized food in my life.
- I've changed the way I think about myself. I now like myself.
- I understand that the changes I am making will become a part of the rest of my life.
- The way I look is very important to me. I always strive to look my best.
- I've learned to see situations as they really are rather than imagining the worst.
- I am confident that I can cope with every circumstance without reverting to food.
- I like me.
- I enjoy my new-found freedom from being overweight.
- I believe in me and what I have set out to accomplish.
- I look forward to rather than dread each new day.
- I see the beauty all around me that I've missed while overeating.
- I appreciate life more.
- My attitude is more positive in all phases of my life.
- I am a success.

A nun once told one of our lecturers that you need three things to be a good nun and a good dieter: a wishbone, a funny bone, and a backbone.

We hope that we have strengthened your "bones." We have now given you the tools to continue the Lean Line One Month Lighter Program one month at a time—for as long as you wish. Now go out and live. The world is waiting for the new you!

PART II

MORE
LEAN
LINE
RECIPES

DRESSINGS, SAUCES, DIPS

▮ LEAN LINE TOMATO SAUCE ▮
35 calories

---

8 oz tomato juice

---

1 clove garlic, minced

Salt, pepper, oregano, basil, onion powder, and garlic powder to taste

---

Combine all ingredients and simmer until thickened, 20–35 minutes, depending on brand of tomato juice used.

COUNTS AS: Daily tomato juice from Free Food List

▎ SALAD DRESSING AND ONION DIP ▎
(2 servings) 50 calories per serving

4 oz (½ cup) low-fat plain yogurt
1 packet onion bouillon powder, undissolved
1 teaspoon onion flakes
½ teaspoon garlic powder
1 teaspoon imitation mayonnaise

Mix together all ingredients.

EACH SERVING COUNTS AS: ½ Milk Selection
¼ Oil and Condiment Selection

▎ BARBECUE SAUCE ▎
(4 servings) 40 calories per serving

16 oz (2 cups) tomato juice
2 oz (¼ cup) chopped celery
1 tablespoon dried oregano
4 oz (½ cup) sliced mushrooms
1 teaspoon salt
¼ teaspoon pepper
1 tablespoon vinegar
1 tablespoon Worcestershire sauce or soy sauce
Sprinkling of minced onion
2 oz (¼ cup) chopped green pepper
Artificial sweetener (to equal sweetness of 4 teaspoons sugar)

Combine all ingredients in saucepan and simmer covered over low heat for about 20 minutes, or until thickened.

EACH SERVING COUNTS AS: ½ Daily tomato juice from Free Food List

▮ PEPPER DIP ▮
Less than 1 calorie per 2-tablespoon serving

1 7½-oz jar water-packed roasted peppers, drained
2 tablespoons wine vinegar
2 tablespoons Dijon mustard
Sprinkling of onion flakes
Artificial sweetener (to equal sweetness of 2 teaspoons sugar)

Blend together all ingredients. Great with celery and pepper strips.

COUNTS AS: Free food
Note: Do not use in place of low-calorie salad dressing in One Month Lighter Program.

▮ ONION DRESSING ▮
15 calories

1 packet onion bouillon powder
8 oz (1 cup) boiling water
1½ tablespoons vinegar
Onion and garlic powder to taste
Artificial sweetener (to equal sweetness of 2 teaspoons sugar)

Dissolve bouillon in water. Add vinegar and seasonings. Chill. Shake well before serving. Keep refrigerated. May be served on any type of salad.

COUNTS AS: Free food

Note: Do not use in place of low-calorie salad dressing in One Month Lighter Program.

❚ RED AND SASSY DRESSING ❚
95 calories per 8 tablespoons

4 oz (½ cup) tomato juice
4 oz (½ cup) unsweetened pineapple juice
1 tablespoon lemon juice
Red pepper, basil, and garlic salt to taste

Combine all ingredients in bottle and shake well. Keep refrigerated.

8 TABLESPOONS COUNT AS: 1 Fruit Selection
½ Daily tomato juice from Free Food List

Note: Do not use in place of low-calorie salad dressing in One Month Lighter Program.

▌ ZERO SALAD DRESSING ▌
Less than 1 calorie per 2-tablespoon serving

1½ teaspoons finely chopped green pepper
1 teaspoon onion powder
1½ teaspoons minced fresh parsley
12 oz (1½ cups) wine vinegar
4 oz (1 small jar) water-packed pimentos, drained
24 oz (3 cups) tomato juice
Artificial sweetener to taste (optional)

Blend together and refrigerate. Use as desired.

COUNTS AS: Free Food
Note: Do not use in place of low-calorie salad dressing in One Month Lighter Program.

▌ CREAM SAUCE FOR VEGETABLES ▌
100 calories

4 oz (½ cup) skim or low-fat milk
2 teaspoons arrowroot
½ teaspoon imitation butter flavoring
⅛ teaspoon dry mustard
Salt and pepper to taste

In saucepan, mix together all ingredients and simmer uncovered until thickened, stirring frequently. Pour over cooked vegetables and serve. If you wish, you may also place vegetables in casserole, pour sauce over all, and bake at 350° for 10 minutes.

COUNTS AS: ⅓ Bread Selection
　　　　　　½ Milk Selection

▮ CURRY SAUCE ▮

(2 servings) 115 calories per serving

4 oz (½ cup) finely chopped onions
2 teaspoons imitation margarine
2 tablespoons flour
1 teaspoon curry powder
Salt and pepper to taste
8 oz (1 cup) skim or low-fat milk
2 oz (¼ cup) sliced mushrooms, freshly cooked or canned

In skillet, brown onions in margarine. Add flour, curry powder, salt, and pepper, stirring constantly. Next, gradually stir in milk. Cook uncovered over low heat until thickened. Then add mushrooms and stir. Pour over fully cooked meat, fish, poultry, or vegetables.

EACH SERVING COUNTS AS: ½ Vegetable List A Selection
½ Bread Selection
½ Milk Selection
½ Oil and Condiment Selection

SOUPS

▌ TOMATO SOUP ▌
(4 servings) 95 calories per serving

1 lb (2 cups) chopped fresh tomatoes
1 teaspoon onion flakes
½ bay leaf
½ teaspoon salt
⅛ teaspoon pepper
4 teaspoons imitation margarine
2 tablespoons flour
16 oz (2 cups) skim milk
Fresh basil to taste

In saucepan, combine tomatoes, onion flakes, bay leaf, salt, pepper, and basil and simmer uncovered for 10 minutes. In large pot, melt margarine over low heat. Add flour to melted margarine and blend. Add milk gradually to flour mixture, stirring constantly until slightly thickened. Remove bay leaf from tomato mixture, and add tomato mixture to milk mixture. Heat thoroughly, but do not boil.

EACH SERVING COUNTS AS: ¼ Bread Selection
½ Milk Selection
½ Oil and Condiment Selection
½ Daily tomato juice from Free Food List

▌ VEGETABLE BEEF SOUP ▌
(8 servings) 75 calories per serving

24 oz (3 cups) vegetable juice cocktail
3 packets beef bouillon powder
24 oz (3 cups) water
2 tablespoons parsley flakes
1 teaspoon onion salt
1 tablespoon seasoning salt
Dash of oregano
Pepper to taste
2 teaspoons soy sauce
8 oz (1 cup) chopped celery
8 oz (1 cup) frozen green beans, thawed
4 oz (½ cup) frozen peas, thawed
4 oz (½ cup) frozen whole-kernel corn, thawed
4 oz (½ cup) frozen lima beans, thawed
4 oz (½ cup) sliced potatoes
1 lb cubed cooked lean beef

Place all ingredients except beef in large saucepan. Bring to boil, reduce heat, and simmer covered until tender, about 30 minutes. Divide soup into 8 equal portions. Add 2 oz cooked beef to each serving before reheating. This dish travels very well in thermos for hot cold-day lunches.

EACH SERVING COUNTS AS: 1 Lunch Protein List A
½ Vegetable List B Selection
3 oz Daily vegetable juice from Free Food List

▮ TURKEY NOODLE SOUP ▮
(4 servings) 430 calories per serving

64 oz (8 cups) water
2 lb (4 cups) sliced fresh mushrooms
8 oz (1 cup) chopped celery
8 oz (1 cup) diced carrots
8 oz (1 cup) diced onions
6 packets chicken bouillon powder
½ teaspoon garlic powder
½ bay leaf
Salt to taste
1 lb (2 cups) diced cooked white turkey meat
12 oz (1⅓ cups) cooked enriched noodles

Combine first 9 ingredients in large saucepan. Bring to boil. Reduce heat, and simmer for 10–15 minutes, or until vegetables are tender. Add turkey. Simmer covered 5 minutes longer, or until meat is heated through. Place 3 oz (⅓ cup) noodles in each of 4 large soup bowls. Pour soup over noodles. Serve hot.

EACH SERVING COUNTS AS: 1 Dinner Protein List B
1 Vegetable List A Selection
1 Bread Selection

▌ LOLLY'S STOP A CHEAT SOUP ▌
(8 servings) 55 calories per serving

24 oz (3 cups) water
3 packets chicken or beef bouillon powder
1 10-oz package frozen cauliflower, thawed, or 1¼ cups fresh cauliflowerets
1 10-oz package frozen spinach, thawed, or 1¼ cups fresh spinach
1 10-oz package frozen broccoli, thawed, or 1¼ cups chopped fresh broccoli
4 oz (½ cup) chopped fresh celery
1 lb (2 cups) canned or fresh sliced mushrooms, undrained
1 lb (2 cups) canned or fresh French-style green beans, undrained
Salt, pepper, oregano, and onion powder to taste

Place water, bouillon, cauliflower, spinach, broccoli, and celery in large soup pot. Bring to boil, reduce heat, and simmer covered until vegetables are tender, about 10 minutes. Add mushrooms, green beans, and seasonings. Continue to simmer until all ingredients are cooked.

EACH SERVING COUNTS AS: Free food

▌ BUTTERMILK SOUP FREEZE ▌
(2 servings) 120 calories per serving

12 oz (1½ cups) buttermilk
8 oz (1 medium) cucumber, peeled and diced
1 hard-boiled egg, finely chopped
1 teaspoon onion powder
¼ teaspoon dry mustard
Paprika and salt to taste
1 tablespoon Worcestershire sauce

Put all ingredients in blender and blend well. Chill at least 30 minutes before serving.

EACH SERVING COUNTS AS: 1 Milk Selection
½ Bonus List A Selection (egg)

▌ CHILLED CREAM OF BROCCOLI SOUP ▌
(2 servings) 75 calories per serving

1 10-oz package frozen broccoli or 1¼ cups chopped fresh broccoli
4 oz (½ cup) water
1 packet bouillon powder
Dash onion powder
Salt to taste
8 oz (1 cup) skim milk

Cook broccoli in ½ cup water. Add bouillon and cook until dissolved. Add onion powder and salt. Chill. Put mixture in blender with skim milk. Blend well and serve.

EACH SERVING COUNTS AS: ½ Milk Selection

Protein

❚ BAKED ORANGE SWORDFISH ❚
(3 servings) 255 calories per serving

---

1 lb fresh or frozen swordfish (will cook down to 12 oz)

¼ teaspoon salt

¼ teaspoon grated orange rind

---

4 oz (½ cup) sugar-free orange soda

---

2 tablespoons chopped fresh parsley

Place swordfish steaks in single layer in shallow baking pan. Sprinkle with salt and orange rind. Add orange soda. Bake in

350° oven (basting once or twice with pan juices) for 30 minutes, or until fish flakes easily. Sprinkle with parsley and serve.

COUNTS AS: 1 Lunch Protein List B

▌CRAB CROQUETTES ▌
(6 servings) 225 calories per serving

1 egg
3 tablespoons sour cream
1½ tablespoons imitation mayonnaise
2 teaspoons prepared mustard
2 teaspoons minced fresh parsley
1 tablespoon minced chives
1½ pounds (3 cups) lump crab meat, cartilage removed
6 oz (6 slices) whole-wheat bread

Beat egg lightly. Stir in sour cream, mayonnaise, mustard, parsley, and chives. Pour mixture over crab meat and mix lightly. Remove crust from bread, press bread into large custard cups, and fill each cup with one-sixth of crab-meat mixture. Bake in 400° oven for approximately 12 minutes, or until bread edges are toasted.

EACH SERVING COUNTS AS: 1 Lunch Protein combined Lists B and C
1 Bread Selection
⅔ Oil and Condiment Selection

▮ GRILLED HADDOCK ▮
480 calories

---

8 oz filet of haddock (will cook down to 6 oz)

Garlic powder, black pepper, and lemon juice to taste

---

4 oz (½ cup) sliced onions

Sliced green pepper (as desired)

---

6 oz (¾ cup) water or 3 oz (⅓ cup) white wine and 3 oz (⅓ cup) water

---

Place haddock on double layer of aluminum foil and sprinkle with garlic powder, pepper, and lemon. Arrange onions and green pepper around fish. Pour water over fish and vegetables. Wrap foil tightly, and grill for approximately 40 minutes.

COUNTS AS: Protein List B
1 Vegetable List A Selection
1 Bonus List B Selection (wine)

▮ LIGHT TUNA CROQUETTES ▮
(2 servings) 185 calories per serving

---

7 oz (⅞ cup) water-packed tuna with 1 tablespoon water-packed tuna liquid

---

1 egg

½ teaspoon prepared mustard

---

1 oz (2 tablespoons) bread crumbs

Combine tuna, tuna liquid, egg, mustard, and half the bread crumbs. Stir well. Make into 4 croquettes. Roll in remaining bread crumbs. Over medium heat, fry croquettes in nonstick skillet or skillet coated with no-stick vegetable cooking spray for 3–4 minutes, or until browned. Turn croquettes over and fry approximately 3 minutes more, or until browned on other side.

EACH SERVING COUNTS AS: 1 Lunch Protein combined
Lists B and C
1 Bread Selection

▌ TUNA REUBEN ▌
330 calories

2 oz (¼ cup) water-packed tuna
2 teaspoons sour cream
⅛ teaspoon onion powder
2 oz (2 slices) bread
1 oz (1 slice) any natural hard cheese

Drain tuna. Add sour cream and onion powder, and mix well.
Toast bread. Put tuna mixture on 1 slice of bread and hard cheese
on other slice of bread. Put under broiler for 2–3 minutes, until
cheese is melted. Make sandwich and serve.

COUNTS AS: 1 Lunch Protein combined Lists B and C
2 Bread Selections
½ Oil and Condiment Selection

▌ TUNA AND EGG CASSEROLE ▌
575 calories

1 egg
4 oz (½ cup) water-packed tuna, crumbled or flaked
6 oz (⅔ cup) cooked flat enriched noodles
4 oz (½ cup) canned or fresh sliced mushrooms
4 oz (½ cup) canned carrots
2 tablespoons imitation mayonnaise
Salt and pepper to taste

Combine all ingredients. Coat baking or casserole dish with no-stick vegetable cooking spray, and bake in 350° oven until edges are bubbling.

COUNTS AS: 1 Dinner Protein List B
1 Vegetable List A Selection
2 Bread Selections
3 Oil and Condiment Selections

▮ SCRAMBLED EGGS WITH CHICKEN BOUILLON AND CHEESE ON TOAST ▮
(4 servings) 215 calories per serving

4 oz (4 slices) natural American or cheddar cheese
8 oz (1 cup) hot chicken bouillon
4 eggs, beaten
1 tablespoon onion powder
1 tablespoon chopped fresh parsley
Grating of nutmeg
¼ teaspoon salt
⅛ teaspoon paprika
4 oz (4 slices) bread, toasted without butter or margarine

Melt cheese in double boiler. Beat together bouillon, eggs, onion powder, parsley, nutmeg, and paprika. Add to melted cheese, and continue cooking, stirring, until ingredients are firm. Divide into 4 portions and serve each portion on 1 slice of toasted bread.

COUNTS AS: 1 Lunch Protein List C
1 Bread Selection

▎ SCRAMBLED EGGS AND CRAB MEAT ▎
(3 servings) 200 calories per serving

6 oz (¾ cup) cooked crab meat
¼ teaspoon curry powder
⅛ teaspoon paprika
3 eggs
2 oz (¼ cup) skim milk
Dash of salt

In nonstick pan or pan coated with no-stick vegetable cooking spray, heat crab meat, curry powder, and paprika. Meanwhile, beat together lightly eggs, milk, and salt. Add egg mixture to crab-meat mixture. Stir gently over medium heat until eggs set.

COUNTS AS: 1 Lunch Protein combined Lists B and C *or* 1 Dinner Protein combined Lists B and C

▎ RICE À LA ESPAGNOL ▎
(2 servings) 215 calories per serving

2 oz (¼ cup) uncooked enriched white rice
6 oz (¾ cup) uncooked lean ground beef (will cook down to 4 oz)
1½ oz (3 tablespoons) chopped onions
½ oz (½ medium) green pepper, chopped
½ oz (1 small) stalk celery, chopped
8 oz (1 cup) canned or chopped fresh tomatoes

Cook rice according to package directions. Place beef in large nonstick frying pan or pan coated with no-stick vegetable cooking spray and fry until browned. Drain off fat. Mix together rice and beef in same pan. Add onions, green pepper, and celery. Stir in tomatoes. Cover, and simmer about 30 minutes, or until rice is tender and all water is absorbed.

EACH SERVING COUNTS AS: 1 Lunch Protein List A
1 Bread Selection
½ Daily tomato juice from Free Food List

∎ ZUCCHINI AND FRANKFURTER DINNER ∎
355 calories

4 oz (½ cup) vegetable juice cocktail
8 oz (1 medium) zucchini, cubed
4 oz (½ cup) canned or fresh sliced mush-rooms, drained
2 oz (1 medium) frankfurter, sliced into ¼-inch slices
Oregano, salt, and pepper to taste
1 oz (1 slice) part-skim mozzarella cheese, grated

Simmer all ingredients except cheese in saucepan. Transfer mixture to small casserole coated with no-stick vegetable cooking spray. Sprinkle with cheese. Bake at 375° for 20 minutes, or until cheese is golden brown.

COUNTS AS: 1 Dinner Protein combined Lists A and C
½ Daily vegetable juice from Free Food List

▋ SPLIT-PEA CASSEROLE ▋
(3 servings) 445 calories per serving

5 oz (1 cup) fresh or canned ground beef or pork
2 oz (¼ cup) uncooked enriched white rice
8 oz (1 cup) canned or chopped fresh tomatoes
½ teaspoon salt
Pepper to taste
3 oz (⅓ cup) water
8 oz (1 cup) cooked split peas

Place meat in nonstick frying pan or pan coated with no-stick vegetable cooking spray. Brown meat over medium heat. Drain off fat. Cook rice according to package directions. Add rice, tomatoes, salt, pepper, and water to meat. Cover and simmer for about 30 minutes, or until rice is tender and all water is absorbed. Add split peas. Heat until warm.

EACH SERVING COUNTS AS: 1 Dinner Protein combined Lists A and D
1 Bread Selection

▋ PEPPERS AND EGGS ▋
200 calories

2 oz (¼ cup) diced green peppers
1 oz (2 tablespoons) diced onions
4 oz (½ cup) water
2 eggs, lightly beaten
Onion powder, salt, and pepper to taste
1 teaspoon butter

Place green pepper and onions in heavy skillet with ½ cup water, and cook uncovered until tender. Add eggs, onion powder, salt, and pepper, and stir. Melt butter in separate skillet over medium heat. Add egg mixture and continue cooking, stirring, until eggs are set.

COUNTS AS: 1 Lunch Protein List C
¼ Vegetable List A Selection
1 Oil and Condiment Selection

▌ VEAL TURNOVERS ▌
335 calories

2 oz (2 slices) bread
2 oz (¼ cup) cooked ground veal
1 oz (1 slice) part-skim mozzarella cheese, grated

Roll each slice of bread thin. Place half of veal on each slice, top with cheese, and fold in half diagonally. Moisten edges of bread and press together with fork. Bake at 350° for 20 minutes.

COUNTS AS: 1 Lunch Protein combined Lists B and C *or* ½ Dinner Protein combined Lists B and C
2 Bread Selections

▌ VEAL-STUFFED CABBAGE ▌
565 calories

4 oz (2 cups) cabbage leaves
6 oz (¾ cup) cooked ground veal
2 oz (½ small) green pepper, diced
4 oz (½ cup) chopped onions
3 oz (⅓ cup) cooked enriched white rice
Salt and pepper to taste
8 oz (1 cup) tomato juice

Parboil cabbage leaves. Mix veal with green pepper, onions, rice, salt, and pepper. Place some mixture in center of each cabbage leaf, fold edges of leaf over mixture, and roll up. Place in baking dish. Pour tomato juice over all and bake at 375° for approximately 30 minutes.

COUNTS AS: 1 Dinner Protein List B
1 Vegetable List A Selection
1 Bread Selection
Daily tomato juice from Free Food List

∎ SWISS TUNA CASSEROLE ∎
570 calories

4½ oz (½ cup) cooked enriched egg noodles
4 oz (½ cup) water-packed tuna
1 oz (1 slice) natural Swiss cheese, grated
2 oz (¼ cup) fresh sliced mushrooms
8 oz (1 cup) skim milk
1 tablespoon flour
Salt and pepper to taste
4 teaspoons sour cream

In bowl, combine noodles, tuna, Swiss cheese, and mushrooms. Turn out into small casserole coated with no-stick vegetable cooking spray. In small saucepan, combine milk, flour, salt, and pepper. Cook until thickened and then add sour cream. Pour milk mixture over noodle mixture. Bake at 350° for 30 minutes.

COUNTS AS: 1 Dinner Protein combined Lists B and C
2 Bread Selections *or* 1 Bread and 1 Bonus List A
1 Milk Selection
1 Oil and Condiment Selection

▌ VEAL QUICHE ▌
395 calories

2 teaspoons imitation margarine
4 oz (2 cups) sliced fresh mushrooms
2 oz (¼ cup) cooked ground veal
4 oz (½ cup) skim milk
1 oz (2 tablespoons) grated Swiss cheese
Salt, pepper, oregano, and garlic powder to taste
1 egg, beaten

In saucepan, melt margarine. Add mushrooms and sauté until soft. Add ground veal, milk, cheese, and seasonings, and mix. Turn out into 1-quart baking dish and top with beaten egg. Bake at 350° for 30 minutes.

COUNTS AS: 1 Lunch Protein combined Lists B and C and ½ Bonus List A Selection *or* 1 Dinner Protein combined Lists B and C
½ Milk Selection
1 Oil and Condiment Selection
1 Bonus List A Selection

▌ SALMON CROQUETTES ▌
165 calories

3 oz (⅓ cup) canned salmon
2 teaspoons dehydrated onion flakes
2 oz (¼ cup) finely diced celery
Prepared mustard to moisten
Horseradish (optional)

Drain and flake salmon. Add onion flakes and celery, then enough mustard to moisten. Shape into patties. Place on foil, and bake at 350° for 20 minutes, or until slightly browned, turning once. Serve with horseradish if desired.

COUNTS AS: 1 Dinner Protein List A

❚ TUNA FISH CHEF'S SALAD ❚
100 calories

4 oz (¼ head) lettuce
3 oz (⅓ cup) water-packed tuna
3–6 fresh mushrooms, sliced thin
½ hard-boiled egg
4 teaspoons low-calorie salad dressing

Break lettuce into bite-sized pieces. Crumble tuna into coarse pieces and scatter over lettuce, along with remaining ingredients. Spoon dressing over salad, toss, and serve immediately.

COUNTS AS: 1 Lunch Protein List B *or* 1 Dinner Protein List B
                1 Oil and Condiment Selection

❚ FLOUNDER STUFFED WITH CRAB MEAT ❚
(3 servings) 365 calories per serving

½ lb (1 cup) cooked crab meat
Salt, pepper, parsley flakes, and onion powder to taste
1 lb (2 medium) flounder filets (cooks down to 12 oz)
Lemon juice and paprika to taste

Combine crab meat and seasonings, and mix well. Spread out flounder filets, place seasoned crab meat on flounder, and roll up, jelly-roll fashion. Secure with toothpicks. Place stuffed flounder in baking pan sprayed with no-stick vegetable cooking spray, sprinkle with lemon juice, and top with paprika. Bake at 400° 15–20 minutes, or until flounder flakes easily with fork.

EACH SERVING COUNTS AS: 1 Dinner Protein List B

▮ CHICKEN LOAF ▮
390 calories

1 envelope unflavored gelatin
8 oz (1 cup) cold chicken bouillon
4 oz (½ cup) buttermilk
2 teaspoons freshly squeezed lemon juice
½ teaspoon grated lemon rind
¼ teaspoon salt
6 oz (¾ cup) diced cooked chicken
4 oz (½ cup) chopped celery
1 tablespoon chopped fresh parsley

In saucepan, sprinkle gelatin over bouillon. Stir over low heat until gelatin dissolves. Remove from heat and stir in buttermilk, lemon juice, lemon rind, and salt. Chill until mixture is consistency of unbeaten egg whites. Fold in chicken, celery, and parsley. Turn out into small loaf pan. Chill until firm. Serve cold.

COUNTS AS: 1 Lunch Protein List B and ½ Bonus List A Selection *or* 1 Dinner Protein List B
¾ Milk Selection

▮ CHICKEN CACCIATORE ▮
475 calories

6 oz boneless chicken (will cook down to 4 oz)
1 oz (2 tablespoons) diced onions
8 oz (2 small) tomatoes, peeled and chopped
3 oz (⅓ cup) home-style meatless oil-free to- mato sauce
4 oz (½ cup) vegetable juice cocktail
Salt, pepper, onion flakes, basil, and oregano to taste
3 oz (1 medium) green pepper, cut into strips
3 oz (⅓ cup) cooked enriched white rice

Broil chicken on rack. Cut into strips. In skillet, combine chicken, onions, tomatoes, tomato sauce, juice, seasonings, and green pepper. Bring to boiling, reduce heat, and simmer for 20 minutes. Serve over rice.

COUNTS AS: 1 Dinner Protein List B
1 Vegetable List A Selection
1 Bread Selection
½ Daily vegetable juice from Free Food List

▮ VEAL-STUFFED EGGPLANT ▮
(2 servings) 380 calories per serving

8 oz (1 medium) eggplant
8 oz (1 cup) Lean Line Tomato Sauce (see page 197)
Salt, pepper, garlic powder, and oregano to taste
12 oz broiled ground veal patty, broken up into pieces

Slice eggplant in half lengthwise and scoop out pulp. In saucepan, cook over medium heat eggplant pulp in tomato sauce with seasonings until tender, but not mushy. Mix ground veal with eggplant. Fill each eggplant shell with half of veal-eggplant mixture. Bake at 350° for about 30 minutes, or until done but not dry.

EACH SERVING COUNTS AS: 1 Dinner Protein List B
½ Daily tomato juice from Free Food List

▌ DALEY'S TACOS ▌
385 calories

2 oz (¼ cup) cooked lean ground beef
Chili, onion, and garlic powders to taste
2 oz (1 large) pita bread, warmed
1 oz (1 slice) natural cheddar cheese, cubed
Lettuce and tomato, chopped (as desired)
4 oz (½ cup) Lean Line Tomato Sauce (see page 197)

In nonstick skillet or skillet coated with no-stick vegetable cooking spray, fry ground beef and drain off fat. Add seasonings. Split pita bread and fill with beef. Top with cheese, lettuce, tomato, and tomato sauce.

COUNTS AS: 1 Dinner Protein List A
2 Bread Selections
½ Daily tomato juice from Free Food List

▌ IMITATION PASTAFOCULE, OR OLLIE'S CASSEROLE ▌
500 calories

½ oz (1 tablespoon) diced onions
4 oz (½ cup) diced green pepper
2 oz (¼ cup) canned vegetarian beans in to-mato sauce
4 oz (½ cup) tomato juice
4 oz (½ cup) water
3 oz (1½ small) hot dogs, sliced
Salt, pepper, and onion powder to taste
3 oz (⅓ cup) cooked elbow macaroni

In large nonstick skillet or skillet coated with no-stick vegetable cooking spray, sauté onions and green pepper until tender. Add beans, tomato juice, water, hot dogs, and seasonings. Cook uncovered for 20 minutes over medium heat, stirring frequently. Add macaroni and mix well. Add more pepper if you like it spicy. Serve warm.

COUNTS AS: 1 Dinner Protein List A
1 Vegetable List B Selection
1 Bread Selection
½ Daily tomato juice from Free Food List

▮ LEAN LINE PASTA LUNCH ▮
500 calories

4 oz carrots
4 oz celery
2 oz (1 medium) frankfurter
4 oz (½ cup) canned or fresh sliced mushrooms
3 oz (⅓ cup) cooked thin spaghetti or other pasta
3 oz (⅓ cup) skim milk
Dash parsley flakes and oregano
Salt and pepper to taste
½ packet Butter Buds
1 oz (2 tablespoons) grated Parmesan cheese

Cut carrots, celery, and frankfurter into matchstick-size strips. In saucepan, boil carrots and celery until tender, about 15–20 minutes. Drain. Place all vegetables, frankfurter, and pasta into saucepan. In small container with airtight lid, combine skim milk, seasonings, and Butter Buds, and shake until well mixed. Add to saucepan mixture and simmer for 5 minutes. Add cheese and toss.

COUNTS AS: 1 Lunch Protein combined Lists A and C
1 Vegetable List A Selection
1 Bread Selection
⅓ Milk Selection

▮ LINGUINE IN CLAM SAUCE ▮
400 calories

6 oz (¾ cup) minced fresh or canned clams
6 oz (¾ cup) reserved clam liquid
2 teaspoons olive oil
1 clove garlic, crushed
1 teaspoon dried oregano
1 tablespoon fresh chopped parsley or dried parsley flakes
Salt and pepper to taste
6 oz (⅔ cup) cooked linguine

Drain clams, reserving liquid, and set aside. In saucepan, combine clam liquid, oil, garlic, oregano, parsley, salt, and pepper. Heat to boiling. Remove from heat and add minced clams. Serve over cooked linguine.

COUNTS AS: 1 Dinner Protein List B
2 Bread Selections
2 Oil and Condiment Selections

▮ MATZO-MEAL PANCAKES ▮
275 calories

1 egg yolk
1½ oz (3 tablespoons) matzo meal
2 oz (¼ cup) cold water
Salt and onion powder to taste
1 egg white, stiffly beaten
1 teaspoon vegetable shortening

Beat together egg yolk, matzo meal, water, salt, and onion powder. Fold in egg white carefully, mixing well. Melt shortening in
nonstick skillet. Drop batter by tablespoonfuls onto skillet and fry
until lightly browned on both sides.

COUNTS AS: 1 Breakfast or ½ Lunch or ⅓ Dinner Protein List
C *or* 1 Bonus List A Selection
2 Bread Selections
1 Oil and Condiment Selection

Note: If served with 4 oz (½ cup) unsweetened applesauce, it
counts additionally as 1 Fruit Selection.

PIZZAS

▮ EASY PIZZA ▮
275 calories

---

2 oz (2 slices) part-skim mozzarella cheese

---

2 oz (¼ cup) Lean Line Tomato Sauce (see page 197)

Oregano, garlic powder, and onion powder to taste

---

1 oz (1 slice) bread

Put mozzarella cheese, tomato sauce, and seasonings on bread. Heat on cookie sheet in 350° oven until cheese melts.

COUNTS AS: 1 Lunch Protein List C *or* ⅓ Dinner Protein List C
1 Bread Selection
¼ Daily tomato juice from Free Food List

▌ MUSHROOM PIZZA ▌
200 calories

1 oz (1 slice) part-skim mozzarella cheese
2 oz (¼ cup) Lean Line Tomato Sauce (see page 197)
2 oz (¼ cup) sliced fresh mushrooms
Oregano, garlic powder, and onion powder to taste
1 oz (1 slice) bread

Put mozzarella cheese, tomato sauce, mushrooms, and seasonings on bread. Heat on cookie sheet in 350° oven until cheese melts.

COUNTS AS: 1 Breakfast Protein List C *or* ½ Lunch Protein List C
1 Bread Selection
¼ Daily tomato juice from Free Food List

▌ HOT-PEPPER PITA PIZZA ▌
310 calories

1 oz (½ large) pita bread
2 oz (2 slices) part-skim mozzarella cheese
1 oz (2 tablespoons) diced hot peppers
1 oz (2 tablespoons) sliced fresh mushrooms
2 oz (¼ cup) Lean Line Tomato Sauce (see page 197)
Oregano, garlic powder, and onion powder to taste

Split pita bread and fill with mozzarella cheese, hot peppers, mushrooms, tomato sauce, and seasonings. Heat in 350° oven on cookie sheet until cheese melts.

COUNTS AS: 1 Lunch Protein List C *or* ⅔ Dinner Protein List C
1 Bread Selection
¼ Daily tomato juice from Free Food List

∎ SAUSAGE PITA PIZZA ∎
255 calories

1 oz (⅛ cup) ground veal
1 oz (½ large) pita bread, split
2 oz (¼ cup) Lean Line Tomato Sauce (see page 197)
1 oz (1 slice) part-skim mozzarella cheese
Oregano, garlic powder, and onion powder to taste

Broil veal on rack until golden brown. Let cool and crumble. Fill pita bread with veal, tomato sauce, mozzarella, and seasonings. Heat in 350° oven until cheese melts.

COUNTS AS: 1 Lunch Protein combined Lists B and C *or* ½ Dinner Protein combined Lists B and C
1 Bread Selection
¼ Daily tomato juice from Free Food List

■ PIZZA POCKET ■
280 calories

2 oz (¼ cup) part-skim ricotta cheese
1 oz (1 slice) part-skim mozzarella cheese, grated
2 oz (½ small) green pepper, diced
4 oz (1 small) tomato, diced
Parsley, garlic salt, garlic powder, oregano, and pepper to taste

Mix together cheese, green pepper, tomato, and seasonings. Split pita and fill with cheese mixture. Stand upright in pan and bake at 400° for 15 minutes.

COUNTS AS: 1 Lunch Protein List C *or* ½ Dinner Protein List C
1 Bread Selection
½ Daily tomato juice from Free Food List

■ PIZZA PUFF ■
(4 servings) 390 calories per serving

4 oz (8 very thin slices) bread
4 oz (½ cup) Lean Line Tomato Sauce (see page 197)
6 oz (6 slices) part-skim mozzarella cheese, sliced into thin strips
6 oz (¾ cup) cooked ground veal
3 eggs
16 oz (2 cups) skim milk
1½ teaspoons fresh or dried basil
Salt to taste

In baking dish coated with no-stick vegetable cooking spray, place half the bread on bottom of pan. Spread with tomato sauce. Put half the cheese on top, then spread veal evenly over cheese. Place remaining cheese over veal and cover with bread. Combine eggs, milk, basil, and salt. Blend well, Pour over casserole. Refrigerate for several hours. Bake, uncovered, at 400° for 45 minutes.

EACH SERVING COUNTS AS: 1 Dinner Protein combined
Lists B and C
1 Bread Selection
½ Milk Selection
½ Daily tomato juice from
Free Food List

▍ VEAL PIZZA ▍
300 calories

6 oz (¾ cup) tomato juice
2 oz (¼ cup) cooked ground veal
1 oz (½ medium) English muffin
Pinch of oregano, salt, pepper, and garlic powder
1 oz (1 slice) part-skim mozzarella cheese

In saucepan, cook down tomato juice until thickened. Place ground veal on English muffin, and cover with thickened tomato juice. Sprinkle with oregano, salt, pepper, and garlic powder. Top with cheese, and heat in 375° oven until cheese is melted.

COUNTS AS: 1 Lunch Protein combined Lists B and C *or* ½
Dinner Protein combined Lists B and C
1 Bread Selection
¾ Daily tomato juice from Free Food List

VEGETABLES

❚ VEGETABLE NOODLE MEDLEY ❚
(2 servings) 300 calories per serving

8 oz (1 cup) hot chicken bouillon
2 oz (¼ cup) chopped onions
6 oz (¾ cup) cubed cooked lean beef
6 oz (⅔ cup) cooked enriched noodles
2 oz (¼ cup) cooked green peas
2 oz (¼ cup) canned tomatoes, with liquid, chopped
¼ teaspoon garlic powder
Salt and pepper to taste

In heavy skillet, combine bouillon and onions. Cover and cook over medium heat until tender. Add remaining ingredients. Continue to cook until thoroughly heated. Serve hot.

EACH SERVING COUNTS AS: 1 Dinner Protein List A
¼ Vegetable List A Selection
¼ Vegetable List B Selection
1 Bread Selection

▌ ASPARAGUS BAKE ▌
220 calories

8 oz (1 cup) chopped cooked asparagus
½ oz (½ tablespoon) bread crumbs
1 egg, beaten
8 oz (1 cup) skim milk
⅛ teaspoon artificial sweetener (or to taste)
Salt to taste

In bowl, combine asparagus, bread crumbs, beaten egg, and milk. Stir well. Add artificial sweetener and salt. Place mixture in baking dish sprayed with no-stick vegetable cooking spray. Bake at 350° until firm, but not dry.

COUNTS AS: 1 Breakfast Protein List C *or* ½ Lunch Protein List C *or* ⅓ Dinner Protein List C
½ Bread Selection
1 Milk Selection

∎ TOMATO AND ZUCCHINI DELIGHT ∎
(2 servings) 100 calories per serving

8 oz (1 cup) canned or fresh tomatoes
8 oz (2 small) zucchini, sliced, or 1 10-oz package frozen sliced zucchini
1½ oz (½ small) onions, chopped
¼ teaspoon salt
Pepper to taste
1 oz (1 slice) bread

In saucepan, combine all ingredients except bread. Cover and simmer until zucchini is tender, about 20 minutes. Tear bread into pieces and add to hot mixture.

EACH SERVING COUNTS AS: ¼ Vegetable List A Selection
½ Bread Selection
½ Daily tomato juice from Free Food List

∎ GLAZED BEETS ∎
(4 servings) 100 calories per serving

1 lb small beets
1 cup reserved beet cooking water
Artificial sweetener (to equal sweetness of 16 teaspoons sugar)
1 teaspoon salt
Dash pepper
4 teaspoons vegetable oil
2 tablespoons freshly squeezed lemon juice
2 tablespoons potato starch or cornstarch
2 tablespoons water

Cook beets in water to cover until tender. Drain, reserving 1 cup of liquid. Slice beets. In saucepan, combine beet liquid, artificial sweetener, salt, pepper, vegetable oil, and lemon juice. Bring to boiling. In small bowl, mix starch with 2 tablespoons water. Add to boiling beet liquid, stirring constantly. Reduce heat and continue boiling for 2 minutes. Add sliced beets and cook for 2 minutes more. Serve immediately, or cool and reheat when needed.

EACH SERVING COUNTS AS: 1 Vegetable List A Selection
¼ Bread Selection
1 Oil and Condiment Selection

▌ ORIENTAL VEGETABLE DINNER ▌
500 calories

1 teaspoon vegetable oil
2 oz (¼ cup) chopped onions
6 oz cooked boneless chicken, cut into strips
1 cup (½ small head) cooked shredded cabbage
2 oz (¼ cup) cooked julienne carrots
1 medium stalk celery, sliced on diagonal
1½ oz (½ medium) green pepper, cut into strips
Dash of ginger
Salt and pepper to taste
½ oz (1 tablespoon) sesame seeds

Heat oil in wok, sauté onions. Add remaining ingredients and stir-fry over medium heat until tender.

COUNTS AS: 1 Dinner Protein List B
1 Vegetable List A Selection
1 Oil and Condiment Selection
1 Bonus List A Selection (sesame seeds)

▮ CARROT AND BUTTERNUT TZIMMES ▮
(4 servings) 45 calories per serving

8 oz (1 cup) sliced carrots
8 oz (1 cup) cubed butternut squash
1 bottle sugar-free diet cherry soda
Dash ground cinnamon

Place carrots in nonstick pan or pan coated with no-stick vegetable cooking spray. Add squash, soda, and cinnamon. Cook, covered, over medium heat until carrots are soft (most of soda will have cooked out).

EACH SERVING COUNTS AS: 1 Vegetable List A Selection

▮ SCHAV ▮
(4 servings) 110 calories per serving

1 quart water
1 teaspoon salt
1 lb (8 cups) chopped fresh spinach
Juice of 2 lemons (about 6 tablespoons)
Artificial sweetener (to equal sweetness of 6 teaspoons sugar)
16 oz (2 cups) low-fat plain yogurt

Combine water and salt in saucepan. Add spinach and lemon juice. Bring to boiling and simmer covered for 10 minutes. Remove from heat; add sweetener. Chill thoroughly. Just before serving, stir in yogurt.

EACH SERVING COUNTS AS: 1 Milk Selection

∎ L.L. CAULIFLOWER AU GRATIN ∎
200 calories

---

1 10-oz package frozen cauliflower or 1¼ cups fresh cauliflower, cooked and drained

---

2 oz (2 slices) natural American or cheddar cheese, diced

---

4 oz (½ cup) sliced fresh mushrooms

---

1 packet onion bouillon powder, undissolved

Mix together all ingredients in baking dish. Cover and heat in 350° oven until cheese has melted. Season with onion powder.

COUNTS AS: 1 Lunch Protein List C *or* ⅔ Dinner Protein List C

∎ BARBECUED POTATOES ∎
80 calories

---

4 oz (½ medium) potato

Onion bouillon powder, undissolved

---

1 teaspoon butter

Scrub potato; do not peel. Cut in half and sprinkle with onion powder. Add butter to each half, join cut ends, and wrap potato in foil. Place on hot coals until cooked (from 20–35 minutes).

COUNTS AS: 1 Vegetable List B Selection
1 Oil and Condiment Selection

❚ CARROT PUFF ❚
45 calories

---

4 oz (½ cup) sliced carrots, cooked and drained

⅛ teaspoon imitation butter flavoring

⅛ teaspoon ground cinnamon

Artificial sweetener (to equal sweetness of 2 teaspoons sugar)

Mash carrots. Add remaining ingredients and mix until well blended. Place in baking dish sprayed with no-stick vegetable cooking spray, and bake at 350° for 20 minutes.

COUNTS AS: 1 Vegetable List A Selection

❚ GRILLED ONIONS ❚
80 calories

---

4 oz (½ cup) sliced onions

---

2 teaspoons imitation margarine

Salt, pepper, and paprika to taste

Sprinkling of Parmesan cheese

Place all ingredients on double layer of aluminum foil and wrap tightly. Heat on grill, approximately 10 minutes on each side.

COUNTS AS: 1 Vegetable List A Selection
1 Oil and Condiment Selection

▮ RATATOUILLE ▮
275 calories

8 oz (1 cup) tomato juice
12 oz (1½ cups) diced peeled eggplant
12 oz (1½ cups) diced zucchini
8 oz (1 cup) sliced fresh mushrooms
3 oz (1 medium) green pepper, diced
4 oz (1 medium) tomato, diced
4 oz (½ cup) sliced onions
½ cup chicken bouillon
½ bay leaf
Dash garlic powder and basil
1 teaspoon salt (or to taste)
½ teaspoon pepper (or to taste)
1 teaspoon chopped fresh parsley

In heat-proof casserole, combine tomato juice, eggplant, zucchini, mushrooms, green pepper, tomato, onions, bouillon, bay leaf, garlic powder, and basil. Simmer, covered, for 30 minutes. Add salt and pepper; sprinkle with parsley. Remove bay leaf. Serve right from casserole.

COUNTS AS: 1 Vegetable List A Selection
Daily tomato juice from Free Food List

▌ SWEET AND SOUR RED CABBAGE ▌
(4 servings) 35 calories per serving

10 oz (4 cups) shredded red cabbage
4 oz (1 medium) apple, peeled, cored, and thinly sliced
Artificial sweetener (to equal sweetness of 2 teaspoons sugar)
½ teaspoon allspice
1 teaspoon salt
5 tablespoons vinegar

Combine all ingredients in saucepan. Cook covered over low heat, stirring occasionally, for 20 minutes.

EACH SERVING COUNTS AS: ¼ Fruit Selection

▌ ZUCCHINI RICE PIE ▌
(4 servings) 300 calories per serving

4 oz (½ cup) finely chopped onions
8 oz (1 cup) sliced fresh mushrooms
12 oz (1 large) zucchini, chopped
½ teaspoon dried basil
½ teaspoon dried oregano
12 oz (1⅓ cups) cooked enriched white rice
5 beaten eggs
4 oz (½ cup) skim milk
2 oz (4 tablespoons) Parmesan cheese

In nonstick saucepan put ¼ cup water and cook onions, mushrooms, zucchini, basil, and oregano uncovered until tender, but not brown. Stir in rice, eggs, milk, and half the cheese. Turn out into 9-in. pie plate coated with no-stick vegetable cooking spray. Sprinkle with remaining cheese. Bake, uncovered, in 350° oven for 25–30 minutes, or until set. Let stand 10 minutes, and serve.

EACH SERVING COUNTS AS: 1 Lunch Protein List C
¼ Vegetable List A Selection
1 Bread Selection
⅛ Milk Selection

▮ EGGPLANT BAKE ▮
425 calories

8 oz (1 small) eggplant, peeled and cubed
4 oz (½ cup) home-style meatless oil-free to-mato sauce
4 oz (½ cup) vegetable juice cocktail
Basil, oregano, salt, and pepper to taste
4 oz (1 small can) whole mushrooms, drained
3 oz (⅓ cup) part-skim ricotta cheese
1 egg
½ oz (1 tablespoon) Parmesan cheese

In large nonstick skillet or skilled coated with no-stick vegetable cooking spray, simmer eggplant, tomato sauce, vegetable juice cocktail, seasonings, and mushrooms until eggplant is soft, about 20–30 minutes. Mix together remaining ingredients with hand mixer. In small casserole coated with no-stick vegetable cooking spray, put half of eggplant mixture, then half of cheese mixture; repeat layers. Bake at 350° for 40–45 minutes.

COUNTS AS: 1 Dinner Protein List C
1 Vegetable List A Selection
½ Daily vegetable juice from Free Food List

❚ ANTIPASTO SALAD UNLIMITED ❚
75 calories

8 oz (1 cup) canned or fresh French-style green beans
2 oz (¼ cup) canned or fresh sliced mushrooms
2 oz (¼ cup) water-packed pimentos
2 oz (¼ cup) red wine vinegar
2 tablespoons fresh or dried oregano
1 clove garlic, crushed
Salt and pepper to taste

Drain string beans, mushrooms, and pimentos. Place in bowl and add vinegar, oregano, garlic, salt, and pepper. Mix well. Chill for 2–3 hours. Remove crushed garlic before serving.

COUNTS AS: Free food

❚ Raw Mushroom Salad ❚
(4 servings) 30 calories per serving

8 oz (3½ cups) fresh mushrooms
4 teaspoons olive oil
Juice of 1 lemon
Coarse salt, freshly ground black pepper, and garlic powder to taste
2 tablespoons chopped fresh marjoram or parsley

Slice mushrooms thinly. Combine oil, lemon juice, salt, pepper, and garlic powder. Mix thoroughly and pour over mushrooms. Sprinkle with marjoram or parsley.

EACH SERVING COUNTS AS: 1 Oil and Condiment Selection

❚ CREAMED CUCUMBERS ❚
55 calories

8 oz (1 medium) cucumber, peeled and sliced
4 teaspoons sour cream
Artificial sweetener to taste

Combine cucumbers, sour cream, and sweetener. Mix well and serve.

COUNTS AS: 1 Oil and Condiment Selection

❚ STIR-FRIED VEGETABLES ❚
(2 servings) 100 calories per serving

4 oz (½ cup) water
1 packet chicken bouillon powder
8 oz (1 cup) thinly sliced zucchini
8 oz (1 cup) thinly sliced green and red peppers, mixed
4 oz (½ cup) thinly sliced carrots
4 oz (½ cup) thinly sliced onions
8 oz (1 cup) sliced fresh mushrooms

In heavy skillet, combine water and bouillon. Place over medium heat and bring to boiling. Add all vegetables, cover, and cook until vegetables are tender-crisp. Stir occasionally, adding more water if needed.

EACH SERVING COUNTS AS: 1 Vegetable List A Selection

▌ BAKED STUFFED POTATO ▌
85 calories

4 oz (½ small) baked potato
1 oz (2 tablespoons) skim milk
1 oz (2 tablespoons) low-fat cottage cheese
Salt, pepper, chives, paprika, and parsley to taste

Cut baked potato in half lengthwise, scoop out potato, and reserve potato shells. Mash potato and beat in skim milk. Then mix in cottage cheese, salt, pepper, and chives. Refill potato shells with mixture and sprinkle with paprika and parsley. Bake at 350° until top is browned.

COUNTS AS: ¼ Dinner Protein List C
1 Vegetable List B Selection
⅛ Milk Selection

▌ CHINESE RADISH SALAD ▌
40 calories

9 oz (24 small) radishes
½ teaspoon salt
2 tablespoons cider vinegar
Dash of cayenne pepper
Artificial sweetener (to equal sweetness of 2 teaspoons sugar)
Shredded lettuce (as desired)

Trim radishes and cut lengthwise into fans. Sprinkle with salt. Let stand 10–15 minutes, then drain off any liquid. Mix together remaining ingredients and pour over radishes. Let stand a few more minutes to develop flavor.

COUNTS AS: Free food

DESSERTS

▮ PEAR-APPLE ICE CREAM DELIGHT ▮
(2 servings) 225 calories per serving

4 oz (1 medium) fresh apple
4 oz (1 medium) fresh pear
1 teaspoon pumpkin-pie spice
2 teaspoons imitation margarine
½ oz (1 teaspoon) chopped walnuts
5 oz frozen dietary dairy dessert

Peel and core apple and pear. Cut into chunks. Combine fruits, pie spice, margarine, and walnuts. Place in baking dish, cover, and bake at 350° for approximately 30 minutes, or until soft. Stir once during baking. Cool slightly. Divide equally into 2 portions and spoon over dietary dessert.

EACH SERVING COUNTS AS: 1 Fruit Selection
1 Milk Selection
1 Oil and Condiment Selection

▌ CHOCOLATE CANDY ▌
260 calories

1 serving low-calorie hot cocoa mix, undissolved

4 oz (½ cup) canned unsweetened crushed pineapple, drained

¾ oz (¾ cup) crispy rice cereal

1 teaspoon peanut butter

Mix together all ingredients. Spread on foil and roll foil tightly. Freeze for 1 hour.

COUNTS AS: 1 Bread Selection
1 Fruit Selection
1 Milk Selection
1 Oil and Condiment Selection

▮ CHAROSES ▮
150 calories

1½ oz (3 tablespoons) red wine
2 teaspoons honey
½ oz (1 tablespoon) chopped walnuts
1 oz (2 tablespoons) chopped apple
Ground cinnamon to taste

Mix together all ingredients.

COUNTS AS: ¼ Fruit Selection
1 Oil and Condiment Selection
1 Bonus List B Selection (wine)

▮ YOGURT AND FRUIT DESSERT ▮
(2 servings) 125 calories per serving

1 envelope unflavored gelatin
1 tablespoon lemon juice
2 tablespoons water
8 oz (1 cup) fresh fruit (blueberries, raspberries, peaches, bananas, etc.)
8 oz (1 cup) low-fat plain yogurt
Artificial sweetener to taste (to equal sweetness of 4–8 teaspoons sugar)

Soften gelatin in lemon juice and water. In double boiler or saucepan with hot water, heat over very low heat, stirring until dissolved. Remove from heat. Add fruit, yogurt, and sweetener. Toss lightly. Transfer to blender or food processor, and blend until smooth. Spoon into 2 serving dishes and chill.

EACH SERVING COUNTS AS: 1 Fruit Selection
1 Milk Selection

▮ FRUIT 'N' CRUNCHY ▮
260 calories

4 oz (½ cup) water-packed peaches
2 tablespoons reserved peach liquid
2 oz (¼ cup) low-fat plain yogurt
¾ oz (¾ cup) bran flakes
1 oz (¼ cup) wheat germ

Drain peaches, reserving liquid. Place fruit in bowl. Stir fruit liquid into yogurt. Spoon mixture over fruit. Combine cereal and wheat germ, and sprinkle over fruit.

COUNTS AS: 1 Breakfast Protein List D
1 Bread Selection
1 Fruit Selection
½ Milk Selection

▮ HAWAIIAN DELIGHT ▮
210 calories

4 oz (½ medium) banana, weighed with skin
2 oz (¼ cup) canned unsweetened crushed or chunk-style pineapple
2 oz (¼ cup) orange juice
½ oz (3 teaspoons) peanut butter
Artificial sweetener (to equal sweetness of 4–6 teaspoons sugar)
1 teaspoon coconut extract

Peel and mash banana with fork. One at a time, add remaining ingredients. Pour mixture into freezer container or bowl. Freeze until mixture is consistency of soft ice cream, approximately 45 minutes.

COUNTS AS: 2 Fruit Selections
3 Oil and Condiment Selections

∎ ZUCCHINI CAKE ∎
(8 servings) 210 calories per serving

4 oz (1 cup) all-purpose flour
2 oz (½ cup) wheat germ
6 oz (¾ cup) buttermilk
1 teaspoon ground cinnamon
½ teaspoon salt
2½ teaspoons baking powder
Artificial sweetener (to equal sweetness of 8 teaspoons sugar)
2 oz (4 tablespoons) chopped pecans
4 oz (8 tablespoons) raisins
8 oz (2 cups) shredded zucchini
1 tablespoon vanilla extract
2 eggs
8 teaspoons vegetable oil

Combine first 9 ingredients. Add zucchini, vanilla, eggs, and oil, and stir until well blended. Turn out into 9- x 13-in. pan coated with no-stick vegetable cooking spray. Bake at 375° for 50–55 minutes.

EACH SERVING COUNTS AS: 1 Breakfast Protein combined Lists C and D
1 Bread Selection
1 Fruit Selection
⅛ Milk Selection
1 Oil and Condiment Selection

▮ OATMEAL SQUARES ▮
220 calories

1 oz (2 tablespoons) uncooked oatmeal
⅓ cup nonfat dry milk
1 tablespoon brown-sugar substitute
Artificial sweetener (to equal sweetness of 4 teaspoons sugar)
Dash salt
⅛ teaspoon ground cinnamon
¼ teaspoon vanilla extract
1 teaspoon vegetable oil
2 tablespoons water

Combine first 6 ingredients in small bowl. Stir in remaining ingredients and mix well. Turn out into nonstick pan or pan coated with no-stick vegetable cooking spray. Bake at 350° for 10–15 minutes. Cut into squares.

COUNTS AS: 1 Bread Selection
1 Milk Selection
1 Oil and Condiment Selection

▌ BANANA 'N' LIME PARFAITS ▌
(4 servings) 25 calories per serving

16 oz (2 cups) water
1 3-in. cinnamon stick
4 whole cloves
1 packet sugar-free lime gelatin
1 tablespoon grated lime rind
1 tablespoon freshly squeezed lime juice
8 oz (1 medium) banana, weighed with peel
4 lime twists

In saucepan, heat 1 cup water with cinnamon stick and cloves. Simmer for 5 minutes. Pour over gelatin in bowl. Stir until dissolved. Add remaining 1 cup water, lime rind, and lime juice. Pour half of mixture into 4 glasses. Chill until firm. Pour remaining half of mixture into bowl placed over ice and water. Beat at high speed with hand mixer until frothy. Peel and dice banana, and fold into beaten mixture. Spoon over 4 set gelatins. Chill at least 2 hours. Garnish with lime twist.

EACH SERVING COUNTS AS: ¼ Fruit Selection

❙ SPICE COOKIES ❙
(24 cookies, or 8 servings) 65 calories per serving

4 tablespoons flour
1½ oz (3 tablespoons) uncooked oatmeal
1 egg
8 teaspoons sour cream
¾ oz (4½ teaspoons) raisins
2 oz (¼ cup) unsweetened applesauce
1½ teaspoons brown-sugar substitute
Cinnamon, salt, ginger, cloves, allspice, nutmeg, and vanilla to taste
1 teaspoon baking powder
½ teaspoon baking soda

Mix together all ingredients. Drop spoonfuls onto nonstick cookie sheet or cookie sheet coated with no-stick vegetable cooking spray. Bake 10–12 minutes at 350°.

3 COOKIES COUNT AS: ⅛ Breakfast Protein List C
½ Bread Selection
¼ Fruit Selection
¼ Oil and Condiment Selection

❙ LEAN LINE JELLY BEANS ❙
0 calories

4 envelopes unflavored gelatin
3 packets any flavor sugar-free gelatin
4 cups boiling water

In large bowl, combine unflavored and flavored gelatin. Add boiling water and stir until dissolved. Pour into large, shallow baking pan. Chill, then cut into squares.

COUNTS AS: Free Food

▮ HOT FUDGE SUNDAE ▮
160 calories

1 serving low-calorie hot cocoa mix, undis-solved
3 teaspoons boiling hot water
2½ oz frozen dietary dairy dessert

Stir together cocoa mix and water to make thick sauce. Pour over dairy dessert.

COUNTS AS: 2 Milk Selections

▮ CHOCOLATE-COVERED BANANA ▮
215 calories

4 oz (½ medium) banana, weighed with peel
1 serving low-calorie hot cocoa mix, undis-solved
½ (1 tablespoon) chopped mixed nuts

Peel banana. Freeze on a stick for 1 hour. Dissolve cocoa mix in enough water to make it creamy. Dip frozen banana in chocolate and roll in chopped nuts. Freeze.

COUNTS AS: 1 Fruit Selection
1 Milk Selection
1 Oil and Condiment Selection

▌ BANANA DESSERT ▌
165 calories

4 oz (½ medium) banana, weighed with peel
2 teaspoons imitation margarine
4 tablespoons brown-sugar substitute
Rum flavoring to taste
Ground cinnamon to taste
2½ oz frozen dietary dairy dessert

Peel and slice banana. On low heat, melt margarine in small non-stick frying pan. Add brown-sugar substitute, and stir. Add banana slices, and stir until glazed. Add rum flavoring, turning banana slices gently. Sprinkle with cinnamon. Place dietary dessert in small dish and top with banana mixture.

COUNTS AS: 1 Fruit Selection
1 Milk Selection
1 Oil and Condiment Selection

▌ MINIATURE RAISIN ROLL-UPS ▌
(32 rolls, or 16 servings) 135 calories per serving

1 8-oz package crescent-shaped rolls
8 oz (1 cup) raisins
Ground cinnamon and artificial sweetener to taste
1 teaspoon vegetable oil

Unroll and separate crescent rolls. Roll out each triangle slightly. Cut into halves, making 2 rolls out of 1. Place ¼ oz (½ tablespoon) raisins mixed with cinnamon and sweetener in middle of roll and brush lightly with vegetable oil. Fold up corners of triangle very tightly. Place on nonstick cookie sheet or cookie sheet coated with no-stick vegetable cooking spray. Bake at 350° for 10–13 minutes, or until golden brown. Sprinkle with additional cinnamon and artificial sweetener while still hot.

2 ROLL-UPS COUNT AS: 1 Bread Selection
1 Fruit Selection

∎ PUMPKIN COOKIES ∎
120 calories

4 oz (½ cup) unsweetened pumpkin
⅓ cup nonfat dry milk
Artificial sweetener (to equal sweetness of 4 teaspoons sugar)
Ground cinnamon or pumpkin-pie spice to taste

Combine all ingredients and drop by tablespoonful onto nonstick cookie sheet or cookie sheet coated with no-stick vegetable cooking spray. Bake at 350° for 15 minutes.

COUNTS AS: 1 Vegetable List A Selection
1 Milk Selection

■ PUMPKIN CHEESE PIE ■
(6 servings) 110 calories per serving

2 eggs
8 oz (2 cups) part-skim ricotta or low-fat cottage cheese
6 oz (¾ cup) skim milk
18 oz (2¼ cups) canned unsweetened pumpkin, not pie filling
1 teaspoon vanilla extract
½ teaspoon salt
½ teaspoon ground nutmeg
Artificial sweetener (to equal sweetness of 8 teaspoons sugar)

Combine all ingredients in blender, and blend until smooth. Turn out into pie pan coated with no-stick vegetable cooking spray. Bake in 350° oven for 1 hour.

EACH SERVING COUNTS AS: 1 Breakfast Protein List C
Bonus List A Selection
¾ Vegetable List A Selection
⅛ Milk Selection

▌ BLUEBERRY MUFFINS ▌
(6 muffins, or 2 servings) 270 calories per serving

2 eggs, beaten
2 oz (2 slices) bread, crumbled in blender
2 teaspoons baking powder
⅔ cup nonfat dry milk
Artificial sweetener (to equal sweetness of 12 teaspoons sugar)
2 teaspoons imitation margarine
4 oz (½ cup) fresh blueberries

Combine all ingredients. Spoon into 6 nonstick muffin tins or muffin tins coated with no-stick vegetable cooking spray. Bake at 350° for 25 minutes.

3 MUFFINS COUNT AS: 1 Breakfast Protein List C *or*
1 Bonus List A Selection
1 Bread Selection
½ Fruit Selection
1 Milk Selection
½ Oil and Condiment Selection

▌ BAKED CUSTARD ▌
160 calories

1 egg, slightly beaten
Artificial sweetener (to equal sweetness of 10 teaspoons sugar)
1 teaspoon vanilla extract
8 oz (1 cup) skim or low-fat milk
½ teaspoon ground nutmeg or cinnamon

Combine egg, sweetener, and vanilla. Slowly add skim milk and blend well. Pour mixture into small baking dish. Sprinkle top with nutmeg or cinnamon. Place baking dish in pan of hot water and place in oven. Bake at 325° for 1 hour, or until mixture doesn't adhere to knife.

COUNTS AS: 1 Breakfast Protein List C
or 1 Bonus List A Selection
1 Milk Selection

▮ PIÑA COLADA ▮
110 calories

4 oz (½ cup) skim milk
2 oz (¼ cup) canned unsweetened crushed pineapple, drained
1 teaspoon coconut extract
½ teaspoon rum extract
Artificial sweetener (to equal sweetness of 2 teaspoons sugar)
3 ice cubes

Blend all ingredients except ice in blender. Then add ice cubes 1 at a time, blending thoroughly.

COUNTS AS: ½ Fruit Selection
½ Milk Selection

▌ FRUIT NOG ▌
(2 servings) 160 calories per serving

⅓ *cup nonfat dry milk*
4 oz (½ cup) orange juice
1 egg
8 oz (1 cup) fresh strawberries, washed, hulled, and sliced
4 oz (½ medium) banana, weighed with peel, sliced
3–4 ice cubes

Combine all ingredients except ice cubes in blender and blend until smooth. Add ice cubes 1 at a time. Blend until crushed. Pour into 2 glasses. Serve immediately. Garnish with whole strawberry or banana wedge saved from ingredients.

EACH SERVING COUNTS AS: 1 Fruit Selection
½ Milk Selection
1 Bonus List A Selection

▌ MAPLE SYRUP SHAKE ▌
160 calories

1 egg
8 oz (1 cup) skim milk
2 teaspoons imitation maple syrup
3 ice cubes

In blender, blend all ingredients except ice cubes. Add ice cubes, 1 at a time, and blend until smooth.

COUNTS AS: 1 Breakfast Protein List C
or 1 Bonus List A Selection
1 Milk Selection

▌ PINK PARFAIT ▌
165 calories

⅓ cup nonfat dry milk

---

3 oz (⅓ cup) sugar-free diet cream soda

---

*4 oz (½ cup) fresh strawberries or frozen un-
sweetened strawberries, thawed*

---

*Artificial sweetener (to equal sweetness of 2
teaspoons sugar)*

½ teaspoon vanilla extract

Combine all ingredients in blender. Blend until smooth.

COUNTS AS: ½ Fruit Selection
1 Milk Selection
3 oz Diet soda toward daily allowance of 24 oz

▌ ICE CREAM SODA ▌
80 calories

---

*2½ oz (1 serving) of frozen dietary dairy des-
sert, any flavor*

---

8 oz (1 cup) sugar-free diet soda, any flavor

Combine dietary dessert and soda, and drink with straw.

COUNTS AS: 1 Milk Selection
8 oz diet soda toward daily allowance of 24 oz

▮ EMERGENCY CHOCOLATE FUDGE ▮
165 calories

*1 serving low-calorie hot cocoa mix, undis-
solved*

*Artificial sweetener (to equal sweetness of 2
teaspoons sugar)*

1½ teaspoons water

½ oz (1 tablespoon) chopped mixed nuts

Mix together all ingredients. Drop onto wax paper and freeze until hard.

COUNTS AS: 1 Milk Selection
1 Oil and Condiment Selection

▮ LEAN LINE JAMAICAN COFFEE ▮
30 calories

*4 oz (½ cup) strong black coffee, regular or de-
caffeinated*

*4 oz (½ cup) sugar-free diet cream soda, un-
chilled*

1½ tablespoons imitation whipped cream

Mix coffee and diet soda in glass. Top with imitation whipped cream. Serve hot.

COUNTS AS: 1 Oil and Condiment Selection
4 oz Diet soda toward daily allowance of 24 oz

INDEX

268 INDEX

Broccoli (*cont.*)
Rice Quiche, 97–98
Soup, Chilled Cream of, 207
Supreme, 64–65
Broiling foods, 35
Brussels sprouts, 167
Business lunch, 131–32
Butternut (squash) and Carrot
Tzimmes, 239

Cabbage, 167
Red, Sweet and Sour, 243
Veal Stuffed, 217–18
Caffeine, 35, 182
Cakes
Coconut-Pineapple Creamy
Cheesecake, 125
Zucchini, 253
Calcium, 176, 189
Calories, 38
counting, 183
see also specific recipe
Candy
Chocolate, 250
Jelly Beans, Lean Line, 256–
57
Carrot(s), 167
and Butternut Tzimmes, 239
Puff, 241
Cauliflower au Gratin, Lean Line,
240
Charoses, 251
Cheese, 168
Chicken
Baked, 112
Breaded, Cutlets, 79–80
Cacciatore, 222
East India, 154
Loaf, 221
Polynesian, 50–51
Polynesian, Kabobs, 164
and Roasted Peppers, 69
Chick-Pea Patties, 129
Chocolate
Candy, 250
Covered Banana, 257
Fudge, Emergency, 265
Chow Mein, 122
Club soda, 35

Coffee
and caffeine, 35, 182
decaffeinated, 35, 38, 182
Jamaican, Lean Line, 265
Condiments, 178–79
Cookies
Oatmeal Squares, 254
Pumpkin, 259
Spice, 256
Cooking, 35
vegetables, 166–67
and vitamins, 184
Corn, 167
Muffins, Lean Line, 82
Cornish Hens, Rock, Lemon
Herbed, 140–41
Crab Croquettes, 210
Cucumbers, Creamed, 246

Desserts, 249–62
Apple Chews, Connie's, 68
Baked Custard, 261–62
Banana Dessert, 258
Banana 'n' Lime Parfaits, 255
Charoses, 251
Chocolate Candy, 250
Chocolate-covered Banana,
257
Chocolate Fudge, Emergency,
265
Coconut-Pineapple Creamy
Cheesecake, 125
Fruit 'n' Crunchy, 252
Hawaiian Delight, 252–53
Hot Fudge Sundae, 257
Jelly Beans, Lean Line, 256–57
Miniature Raisin Roll-ups,
258–59
Oatmeal Squares, 254
Pear-Apple Ice Cream Delight,
249–50
Pumpkin Cheese Pie, 260
Pumpkin Cookies, 259
Spice Cookies, 256
Strawberry Rhubarb, 161
Yogurt and Fruit Dessert, 251
Zucchini Cake, 253
see also Muffins
Dinners, *see* Meals; specific recipe